Dash Diet Slow Cooker Beef, Pork & Lamb Cookbook

New Ideas for Tasty Meals

Carmela Rojas

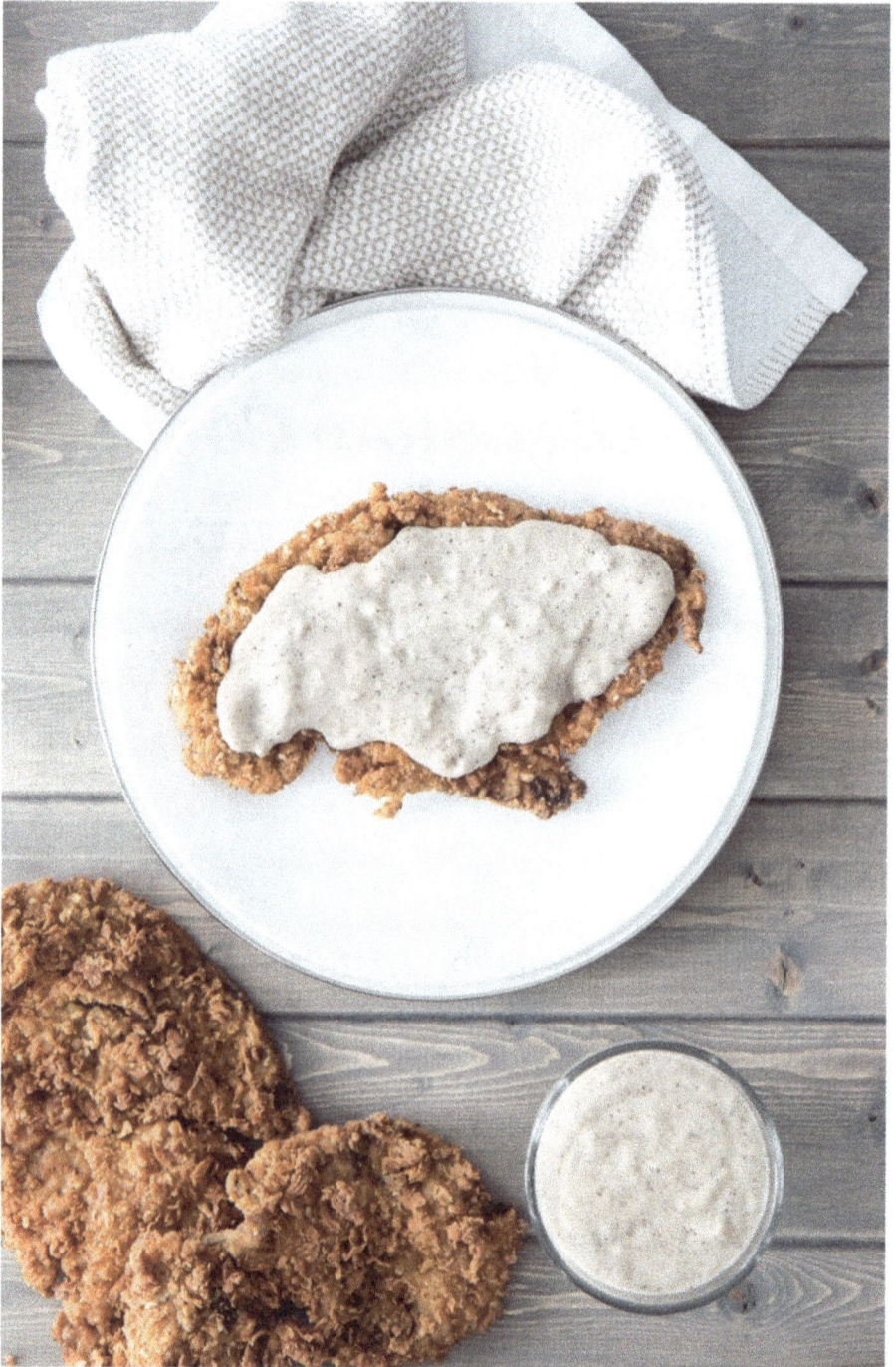

indirect, which are incurred as a result of the use of information contained within this document, including, but not limited to, — errors, omissions, or inaccuracies.

Table of Contents

Smothered Steak

Servings: 6 Servings

Ingredients:

- 2 pounds (900 g) beef round steak
- 2 tablespoons (15 g) onion soup mix
- ¼ cup (60 ml) water
- 10 ounces (280 g) cream of mushroom soup

Directions:

1. Cut steak into 5 to 6 serving-size pieces. Place in slow cooker. Add dry onion soup mix, water, and soup. Cover and cook for 6 to 8 hours.

Nutrition Info:

Per serving: 159 g water; 220 calories (25% from fat, 67% from protein, 9% from carb); 35 g protein; 6 g total fat; 2 g saturated fat; 2 g monounsaturated fat; 0 g polyunsaturated fat; 5 g carb; 0 g fiber; 1 g sugar; 355 mg phosphorus; 13 mg calcium; 3 mg iron; 264 mg sodium; 756 mg potassium; 4 IU vitamin A; 1 mg ATE vitamin E; 0 mg vitamin C; 88 mg cholesterol

Pork For Sandwiches

Servings: 12 Servings

Ingredients:

- 3 pounds (1 1/3 kg) boneless pork shoulder
- 1 large sweet onion, chopped
- 1 tablespoon (10 g) minced garlic
- 1½ cups (413 g) chili sauce
- 2 tablespoons (26 g) sugar
- 2 tablespoons (28 ml) cider vinegar
- 1 tablespoon (15 ml) Worcestershire sauce
- 1 tablespoon (7.5 g) chili powder
- ½ teaspoon black pepper

Directions:

1. Trim fat from pork. If necessary, cut pork to fit slow cooker. Place pork, onion, and garlic in slow cooker. In a medium bowl, combine chili sauce, brown sugar, cider vinegar, Worcestershire sauce, chili powder, and pepper. Pour over pork in cooker. Cover and cook on low for 10 to 11 hours or on high for 5 to 6 hours. Remove park from cooker, reserving juices. Using two forks, shred pork, discarding any fat. Skim

fat from juices. Add enough juices to the pork to moisten.

Nutrition Info:

Per serving: 123 g water; 189 calories (35% from fat, 50% from protein, 14% from carb); 23 g protein; 7 g total fat; 2 g saturated fat; 3 g monounsaturated fat; 1 g polyunsaturated fat; 7 g carb; 1 g fiber; 4 g sugar; 256 mg phosphorus; 19 mg calcium; 2 mg iron; 134 mg sodium; 434 mg potassium; 649 IU vitamin A; 2 mg ATE vitamin E; 10 mg vitamin C; 74 mg cholesterol

Cranberry Pork Roast

Servings: 9 Servings

Ingredients:

- 3 pounds (1 1/3 kg) pork loin roast
- ¼ teaspoon black pepper
- 1 pound (455 g) whole berry cranberry sauce
- ¼ cup (85 g) honey
- 1 teaspoon grated orange peel
- 1/8 teaspoon cloves
- 1/8 teaspoon nutmeg

Directions:

1. Cut roast in half and place in a slow cooker; sprinkle with pepper. Combine the remaining ingredients; pour over roast. Cover and cook on low for 4 to 5 hours or until a meat thermometer reads 160°F (71°C). Let stand 10 minutes before slicing.

Nutrition Info:

Per serving: 144 g water; 299 calories (20% from fat, 43% from protein, 37% from carb); 32 g protein; 6 g total fat; 2 g saturated fat; 3 g monounsaturated fat; 1 g polyunsaturated fat; 27 g carb;

1 g fiber; 27 g sugar; 333 mg phosphorus; 23 mg calcium; 1 mg iron; 92 mg sodium; 579 mg potassium; 33 IU vitamin A; 3 mg ATE vitamin E; 3 mg vitamin C; 95 mg cholesterol

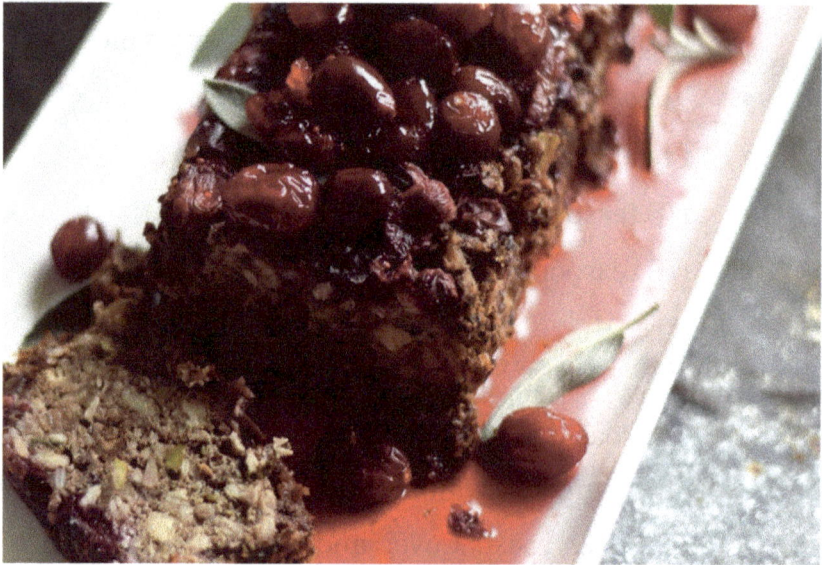

Pan-asian Pot Roast

Servings: 10 Servings

Ingredients:

- 3 pounds (1 1/3 kg) beef chuck roast
- ½ cup (120 ml) orange juice
- 3 tablespoons (45 ml) low-sodium soy sauce
- 2 tablespoons (30 g) brown sugar
- 1 teaspoon Worcestershire sauce

Directions:

1. Place meat in slow cooker. In a mixing bowl, combine remaining ingredients and pour over meat. Cover and cook on low for 8 to 10 hours or on high for 5 hours.

Nutrition Info:

Per serving: 94 g water; 305 calories (32% from fat, 62% from protein, 6% from carb); 45 g protein; 10 g total fat; 4 g saturated fat; 4 g monounsaturated fat; 0 g polyunsaturated fat; 4 g carb; 0 g fiber; 3 g sugar; 372 mg phosphorus; 17 mg calcium; 5 mg iron; 111 mg sodium; 439 mg potassium; 10 IU vitamin A; 0 mg ATE vitamin E; 5 mg vitamin C; 137 mg cholesterol

Short Ribs

Servings: 8 Servings

Ingredients:

- 2/3 cup (83 g) flour
- ½ teaspoon pepper
- 4 pounds (1.8 kg) beef short ribs
- ¼ cup (60 ml) olive oil
- 1 cup (160 g) chopped onion
- 1½ cups (355 ml) low-sodium beef broth
- ½ cup (120 ml) dry red wine
- ¼ cup (60 g) brown sugar
- ½ cup (140 g) chili sauce
- ½ cup (120 g) low-sodium ketchup
- ¼ cup (60 ml) Worcestershire sauce
- 1½ teaspoons minced garlic

Directions:

1. Combine flour and pepper in a plastic bag. Add ribs and shake to coat. Heat half of the oil in a skillet over medium-high heat. Brown half the short ribs and transfer to slow cooker; repeat with remaining oil and meat. Combine remaining ingredients in skillet.

Cook, scraping up browned bits, until mixture comes to boil. Pour over ribs. Cover and cook on low 9 to 10 hours.

Nutrition Info:

Per serving: 260 g water; 567 calories (50% from fat, 33% from protein, 17% from carb); 46 g protein; 30 g total fat; 11 g saturated fat; 15 g monounsaturated fat; 2 g polyunsaturated fat; 24 g carb; 1 g fiber; 12 g sugar; 473 mg phosphorus; 41 mg calcium; 6 mg iron; 267 mg sodium; 1037 mg potassium; 405 IU vitamin A; 0 mg ATE vitamin E; 20 mg vitamin C; 134 mg cholesterol

French Dip

Servings: 12 Servings

Ingredients:
- 3 pounds (1 1/3 kg) beef round roast
- 2 cups (475 ml) low-sodium beef broth
- 2 tablespoons (15 g) onion soup mix
- 12 ounces (355 ml) beer

Directions:
1. Place roast in a slow cooker. Add the beef broth, onion soup, and beer. Cook on low for 7 hours. Slice the meat on the diagonal to serve.

Nutrition Info:

Per serving: 148 g water; 160 calories (26% from fat, 71% from protein, 3% from carb); 26 g protein; 4 g total fat; 1 g saturated fat; 2 g monounsaturated fat; 0 g polyunsaturated fat; 1 g carb; 0 g fiber; 0 g sugar; 255 mg phosphorus; 27 mg calcium; 2 mg iron; 95 mg sodium; 439 mg potassium; 0 IU vitamin A; 0 mg ATE vitamin E; 0 mg vitamin C; 57 mg cholesterol

Italian Roast with Vegetables

Servings: 8 Servings

Ingredients:

- 4 medium potatoes, cut into quarters
- 2 cups (260 g) sliced carrots
- 1 cup (100 g) celery, cut into 1-inch (2.5 cm) pieces
- ½ cup (90 g) diced roma tomato
- 2½ pounds (1.1 kg) beef bottom round roast
- ½ teaspoon black pepper
- 1 can (8 ounces, or 225 g) no-salt-added tomato sauce
- ½ cup (120 ml) water
- 1 tablespoon (10 g) chopped roasted or fresh garlic
- 1 teaspoon basil
- 1 teaspoon oregano
- 1 teaspoon parsley flakes
- 1 teaspoon vinegar

Directions:

1. Place potatoes, carrots, celery, and tomato in slow cooker. Season roast with pepper and place on top. Mix tomato sauce, water, garlic, basil, oregano,

parsley, and vinegar. Pour over roast in cooker. Cover and cook on low 10 to 12 hours or until done.

Nutrition Info:

Per serving: 313 g water; 580 calories (43% from fat, 32% from protein, 25% from carb); 45 g protein; 28 g total fat; 11 g saturated fat; 12 g monounsaturated fat; 1 g polyunsaturated fat; 36 g carb; 5 g fiber; 5 g sugar; 388 mg phosphorus; 69 mg calcium; 5 mg iron; 115 mg sodium; 1443 mg potassium; 5649 IU vitamin A; 0 mg ATE vitamin E; 24 mg vitamin C; 135 mg cholesterol

Honey Mustard Ribs

Servings: 8 Servings

Ingredients:

- 3½ pounds (1.6 kg) country style pork ribs
- 1 cup (250 g) barbecue sauce
- ½ cup (88 g) honey mustard
- 2 teaspoons Salt-Free Seasoning Blend

Directions:

1. Place ribs in a slow cooker. In a small bowl, stir together barbecue sauce, honey mustard, and seasoning blend. Pour over ribs in cooker; stir to coat. Cover and cook on low for 8 to 10 hours or on high for 4 to 5 hours. Transfer ribs to a serving platter. Strain sauce into a bowl; skim fat from sauce. Drizzle some of the sauce over the ribs and pass the remaining sauce at the table.

Nutrition Info:

Per serving: 174 g water; 385 calories (41% from fat, 42% from protein, 17% from carb); 39 g protein; 17 g total fat; 6 g saturated fat; 8 g monounsaturated fat; 2 g polyunsaturated fat;

16 g carb; 0 g fiber; 12 g sugar; 395 mg phosphorus; 54 mg calcium; 2 mg iron; 333 mg sodium; 695 mg potassium; 25 IU vitamin A; 4 mg ATE vitamin E; 2 mg vitamin C; 127 mg cholesterol

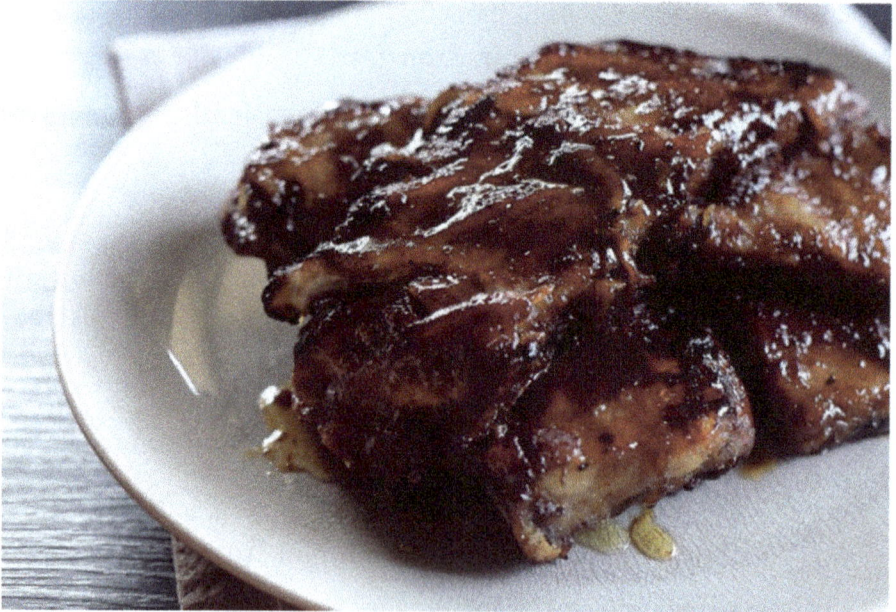

Pizza Casserole

Servings: 6 Servings

Ingredients:

- 1 pound (455 g) sausage
- 1 cup (160 g) chopped onion
- 1 pound (455 g) uncooked pasta
- 28 ounces (785 g) low-sodium spaghetti sauce
- 2 cups (490 g) no-salt-added tomato sauce
- ¾ cup (175 ml) water
- 4 ounces (115 g) mushrooms, sliced
- 4 ounces (115 g) pepperoni
- 2 cups (230 g) shredded mozzarella

Directions:

1. Brown sausage and onion in skillet. Drain. Place half of mixture in slow cooker. Spread half the pasta over the sausage mixture. Combine sauces, water, and mushrooms. Ladle half over pasta. Repeat layers. Top with pepperoni, then cheese. Cover and cook on low 6 to 8 hours.

Nutrition Info:

Per serving: 289 g water; 815 calories (42% from fat, 15% from protein, 43% from carb); 30 g protein; 38 g total fat; 12 g saturated fat; 19 g monounsaturated fat; 4 g polyunsaturated fat; 88 g carb; 8 g fiber; 23 g sugar; 391 mg phosphorus; 87 mg calcium; 4 mg iron; 1025 mg sodium; 1296 mg potassium; 1075 IU vitamin A; 0 mg ATE vitamin E; 27 mg vitamin C; 81 mg cholesterol

Hawaiian Pork Roast

Servings: 4 Servings

Ingredients:

- 1½ pounds (680 g) pork loin roast
- 1 cup (235 ml) pineapple juice
- ¼ cup (60 ml) sherry
- 2 tablespoons (28 ml) low-sodium soy sauce
- 1 teaspoon ground ginger
- 1 tablespoon (13 g) sugar

Directions:

1. Place pork in slow cooker. Combine remaining ingredients and pour over pork. Cover and cook on low until done, but not dry, 4 to 5 hours.

Nutrition Info:

Per serving: 195 g water; 292 calories (24% from fat, 54% from protein, 21% from carb); 37 g protein; 7 g total fat; 2 g saturated fat; 3 g monounsaturated fat; 1 g polyunsaturated fat; 14 g carb; 0 g fiber; 11 g sugar; 387 mg phosphorus; 33 mg calcium; 2 mg iron; 114 mg sodium; 745 mg potassium; 16 IU vitamin A; 3 mg ATE vitamin E; 8 mg vitamin C; 107 mg cholesterol

Apple Cranberry Pork Roast

Servings: 8 Servings

Ingredients:

- 1 tablespoon (15 ml) canola oil
- 3 pounds (1 1/3 kg) pork loin roast
- 2 cups (475 ml) apple juice
- 3 cups (330 g) sliced apples
- 1 cup (100 g) cranberries
- ¼ teaspoon black pepper

Directions:

1. Heat oil in a skillet over medium-high heat. Brown roast on all sides. Place in slow cooker. Add remaining ingredients. Cover and cook on low 6 to 8 hours.

Nutrition Info:

Per serving: 225 g water; 288 calories (29% from fat, 51% from protein, 20% from carb); 36 g protein; 9 g total fat; 3 g saturated fat; 4 g monounsaturated fat; 1 g polyunsaturated fat; 14 g carb; 1 g fiber; 11 g sugar; 381 mg phosphorus; 29 mg calcium; 2 mg

iron; 91 mg sodium; 754 mg potassium; 36 IU vitamin A; 3 mg ATE vitamin E; 5 mg vitamin C; 107 mg cholesterol

Swiss Steak

Servings: 6 Servings

Ingredients:

- ¼ cup (31 g) flour
- 2 pounds (900 g) round steak
- 2 tablespoons (28 ml) olive oil
- 1 cup (160 g) sliced onion
- 1 cup (150 g) green bell pepper strips
- ½ cup (65 g) sliced carrots
- ½ cup (50 g) chopped celery
- 1 teaspoon finely minced garlic
- 1½ cups (355 ml) low-sodium beef broth
- 2 cups (360 g) no-salt-added diced tomatoes, drained
- 1 tablespoon (15 g) brown sugar

Directions:

1. Put the flour in a flat dish. Pound the meat using a meat tenderizer for a few minutes and then dredge the meat in the flour and pound it in. Heat oil in a

large skillet. Add the meat and brown on both sides. Remove the meat from the skillet and add it to your slow cooker. Add the onions, green pepper, carrots, and celery to the skillet and brown. Put them into your slow cooker. Add the beef broth to the skillet and cook over medium heat, scraping the bottom to get all the browned bits. Add this to your cooker along with the tomatoes and brown sugar. Cook on low for 8 to 10 hours.

Nutrition Info:

Per serving: 324 g water; 433 calories (35% from fat, 51% from protein, 14% from carb); 54 g protein; 17 g total fat; 5 g saturated fat; 8 g monounsaturated fat; 1 g polyunsaturated fat; 15 g carb; 2 g fiber; 7 g sugar; 377 mg phosphorus; 60 mg calcium; 6 mg iron; 151 mg sodium; 777 mg potassium; 2017 IU vitamin A; 0 mg ATE vitamin E; 30 mg vitamin C; 157 mg cholesterol

Lamb Cassoulet

Servings: 6 Servings

Ingredients:

- 2 cups (364 g) great northern beans, cooked or canned without salt
- 1 cup (235 ml) dry white wine
- 1 cup (245 g) no-salt-added tomato sauce
- 2 bay leaves
- ½ teaspoon minced garlic
- 1 tablespoon (4 g) fresh parsley
- ½ teaspoon thyme, crushed
- 2 tablespoons (28 ml) olive oil
- 8 ounces (225 g) lean lamb, cut in
- ½-inch (1.3 cm) pieces
- ¾ cup (120 g) chopped onion
- ¼ cup (60 ml) cold water
- 2 tablespoons (16 g) flour

Directions:

1. In a slow cooker combine beans, wine, tomato sauce, bay leaves, garlic, parsley, and thyme. Heat oil in a saucepan over medium-high heat and cook lamb

and onion until lamb is well browned on all sides; drain. Stir lamb and onion into bean mixture in slow cooker. Cover and cook on low for 5 to 6 hours. Turn to high. Heat until bubbly (do not lift cover). Slowly blend the cold water into flour; stir into meat-bean mixture. Cover and cook until slightly thickened. Before serving, remove bay leaves and discard.

Nutrition Info:

Per serving: 181 g water; 274 calories (28% from fat, 29% from protein, 42% from carb); 18 g protein; 8 g total fat; 2 g saturated fat; 4 g monounsaturated fat; 1 g polyunsaturated fat; 26 g carb; 5 g fiber; 3 g sugar; 232 mg phosphorus; 68 mg calcium; 3 mg iron; 40 mg sodium; 638 mg potassium; 187 IU vitamin A; 0 mg ATE vitamin E; 9 mg vitamin C; 34 mg cholesterol

Swiss Steak In Wine Sauce

Servings: 6 Servings

Ingredients:

- For Steak:
- 2 pounds (900 g) beef round steak
- 2 tablespoons (15 g) flour
- ½ teaspoon black pepper
- 2 tablespoons (28 ml) olive oil
- 1 cup (160 g) chopped onion
- ½ cup (65 g) sliced carrot
- 1 can (14 ounces, or 400 g) no-salt-added diced tomatoes
- ¾ cup (175 ml) dry red wine
- ½ teaspoon minced garlic
- For Wine Sauce:
- ¼ cup (60 ml) water
- 2 tablespoons (16 g) flour

Directions:

1. To make the steak: Trim fat from steak; cut meat into 6 equal pieces. Combine flour and pepper and coat meat with mixture. Pound steak to ½-inch (3

cm) thickness using a meat mallet. Heat oil in a large skillet and brown meat; drain. Place onion and carrot in cooker. Place meat on top. Combine undrained tomatoes, wine, and garlic. Pour over meat. Cover and cook on low for 8 to 10 hours. Transfer meat and vegetables to serving platter. Reserve 1½ cups (355 ml) of the cooking liquid for the wine sauce.

2.   To make the wine sauce: Pour reserved liquid into saucepan. Blend cold water slowly into flour; stir into liquid. Cook and stir until thickened and bubbly. Spoon some sauce over meat to serve; pass the remaining sauce at the table.

Nutrition Info:

Per serving: 239 g water; 303 calories (32% from fat, 52% from protein, 16% from carb); 36 g protein; 10 g total fat; 2 g saturated fat; 5 g monounsaturated fat; 1 g polyunsaturated fat; 11 g carb; 2 g fiber; 3 g sugar; 368 mg phosphorus; 39 mg calcium; 4 mg iron; 97 mg sodium; 823 mg potassium; 1872 IU vitamin A; 0 mg ATE vitamin E; 9 mg vitamin C; 86 mg cholesterol

Italian Pork Chops

Servings: 4 Servings

Ingredients:

- 4 boneless pork loin chops
- 1 can (8 ounces, or 225 g) no-salt-added tomato sauce
- 2 tablespoons (15 g) Italian dressing mix
- ¼ cup (60 g) brown sugar
- ¼ cup (44 g) Dijon mustard

Directions:

1. Place pork chops in slow cooker. Mix remaining ingredients together in a bowl. Pour over chops. Cover and cook on low 6 to 8 hours or until meat is tender but not dry.

Nutrition Info:

Per serving: 137 g water; 212 calories (21% from fat, 43% from protein, 35% from carb); 23 g protein; 5 g total fat; 2 g saturated fat; 2 g monounsaturated fat; 1 g polyunsaturated fat; 18 g carb; 1 g fiber; 16 g sugar; 257 mg phosphorus; 41 mg calcium; 2 mg

iron; 233 mg sodium; 652 mg potassium; 214 IU vitamin A; 2 mg ATE vitamin E; 9 mg vitamin C; 64 mg cholesterol

Italian Pot Roast

Servings: 9 Servings

Ingredients:

- 3 pounds (1 1/3 kg) beef round roast
- 2 tablespoons (15 g) Italian dressing mix
- 2 onions, cut in wedges
- ½ teaspoon minced garlic
- 2 cups (300 g) red bell peppers, cut into 1½-inch (3.8 cm) pieces
- ½ cup (120 ml) low-sodium beef broth
- 1 cup (115 g) zucchini, cut into ¼-inch (66 mm) thick slices

Directions:

1. Press dressing mix evenly onto all surfaces of beef roast. Place onions and garlic in slow cooker; top with pot roast. Add red peppers and broth. Cover and cook on high 5 hours or on low 8 hours. Add zucchini. Continue cooking, covered, 30 minutes or until pot roast is tender.

Nutrition Info:

Per serving: 199 g water; 220 calories (24% from fat, 65% from protein, 11% from carb); 35 g protein; 6 g total fat; 2 g saturated fat; 2 g monounsaturated fat; 0 g polyunsaturated fat; 6 g carb; 1 g fiber; 3 g sugar; 354 mg phosphorus; 45 mg calcium; 3 mg iron; 106 mg sodium; 712 mg potassium; 1065 IU vitamin A; 0 mg ATE vitamin E; 47 mg vitamin C; 76 mg cholesterol

Beef With Horseradish Sauce

Servings: 8 Servings

Ingredients:

- 2 tablespoons (28 ml) olive oil
- 3 pounds (1 1/3 kg) beef chuck roast
- ½ teaspoon black pepper
- 1 cup (160 g) chopped onion
- 1 can (6 ounces, or 170 g) no-salt-added tomato paste
- 1/3 cup (85 g) horseradish sauce

Directions:

1. Heat oil in a skillet over medium-high heat; brown roast on all sides. Place in slow cooker. Combine remaining ingredients and pour over roast. Cover and cook on low 8 to 10 hours.

Nutrition Info:

Per serving: 141 g water; 418 calories (37% from fat, 57% from protein, 7% from carb); 57 g protein; 16 g total fat; 5 g saturated fat; 8 g monounsaturated fat; 1 g polyunsaturated fat; 7 g carb; 2 g fiber; 4 g sugar; 483 mg phosphorus; 34 mg calcium; 7 mg

iron; 165 mg sodium; 763 mg potassium; 325 IU vitamin A; 0 mg ATE vitamin E; 9 mg vitamin C; 172 mg cholesterol

Oriental Pot Roast

Servings: 8 Servings

Ingredients:

- 3 pounds (1 1/3 kg) beef chuck roast
- 2 tablespoons (28 ml) olive oil
- 1 pound (455 g) bean sprouts, rinsed and drained
- 5 ounces (140 g) water chestnuts, drained and thinly sliced
- 1 cup (150 g) green bell pepper, cut in 1-inch (2.5 cm) pieces
- 1/3 cup (107 g) apricot jam
- ¼ cup (60 ml) cider vinegar
- 1 tablespoon (15 ml) low-sodium soy sauce
- ½ teaspoon minced garlic
- ½ teaspoon ground ginger
- ¼ teaspoon pepper
- 11 ounces (310 g) mandarin oranges, packed in syrup
- 3 tablespoons (24 g) cornstarch

Directions:

1. Trim excess fat from roast; cut in half to fit into slow cooker. Heat the oil in a skillet over medium-high heat; brown meat and drain. Place meat in cooker; add bean sprouts, water chestnuts, and green pepper. Stir together jam, vinegar, soy sauce, garlic, ginger, and pepper. Pour over meat and vegetables. Cover; cook on low for 8 to 10 hours. Remove meat and vegetables. Skim fat from cooking liquid. Measure 2 cups (475 ml) liquid; reserve. Return meat and vegetables to cooker; cover to keep warm. Drain oranges, reserving ¼ cup (60 ml) of the syrup. In a saucepan, blend reserved syrup slowly into cornstarch; stir in reserved cooking liquid. Cook and stir until thickened and bubbly. Stir in orange sections; heat through. Season to taste. Place meat and vegetables on platter. Spoon some sauce over; pass remaining sauce at the table.

Nutrition Info:

Per serving: 232 g water; 481 calories (32% from fat, 49% from protein, 19% from carb); 58 g protein; 16 g total fat; 5 g saturated fat; 8 g monounsaturated fat; 1 g polyunsaturated fat; 22 g carb; 2 g fiber; 12 g sugar; 499 mg phosphorus; 35 mg calcium; 7 mg iron; 208 mg sodium; 717 mg potassium; 409 IU vitamin A; 0 mg ATE vitamin E; 31 mg vitamin C; 172 mg cholesterol

Barbecued Ribs

Servings: 8 Servings

Ingredients:

- 4 pounds (1.8 kg) pork back ribs
- 2 cups (480 g) low-sodium ketchup
- 1 cup (275 g) chili sauce
- ½ cup (115 g) packed brown sugar
- ¼ cup (60 ml) cider vinegar
- 2 teaspoons oregano
- 2 teaspoons Worcestershire sauce
- 1 dash hot pepper sauce

Directions:

1. Preheat oven to 400°F (200°C, or gas mark 6). Place ribs in a shallow baking pan. Brown in oven 15 minutes. Turn over and brown another 15 minutes; drain fat. In a medium bowl, mix together the ketchup, chili sauce, brown sugar, vinegar, oregano, Worcestershire sauce, and hot pepper sauce. Place ribs in slow cooker. Pour sauce over ribs and turn to coat. Cover and cook on low 6 to 8 hours or until ribs are tender.

Nutrition Info:

Per serving: 211 g water; 766 calories (64% from fat, 20% from protein, 17% from carb); 38 g protein; 54 g total fat; 20 g saturated fat; 24 g monounsaturated fat; 5 g polyunsaturated fat; 32 g carb; 0 g fiber; 29 g sugar; 350 mg phosphorus; 106 mg calcium; 3 mg iron; 224 mg sodium; 825 mg potassium; 1103 IU vitamin A; 7 mg ATE vitamin E; 18 mg vitamin C; 184 mg cholesterol

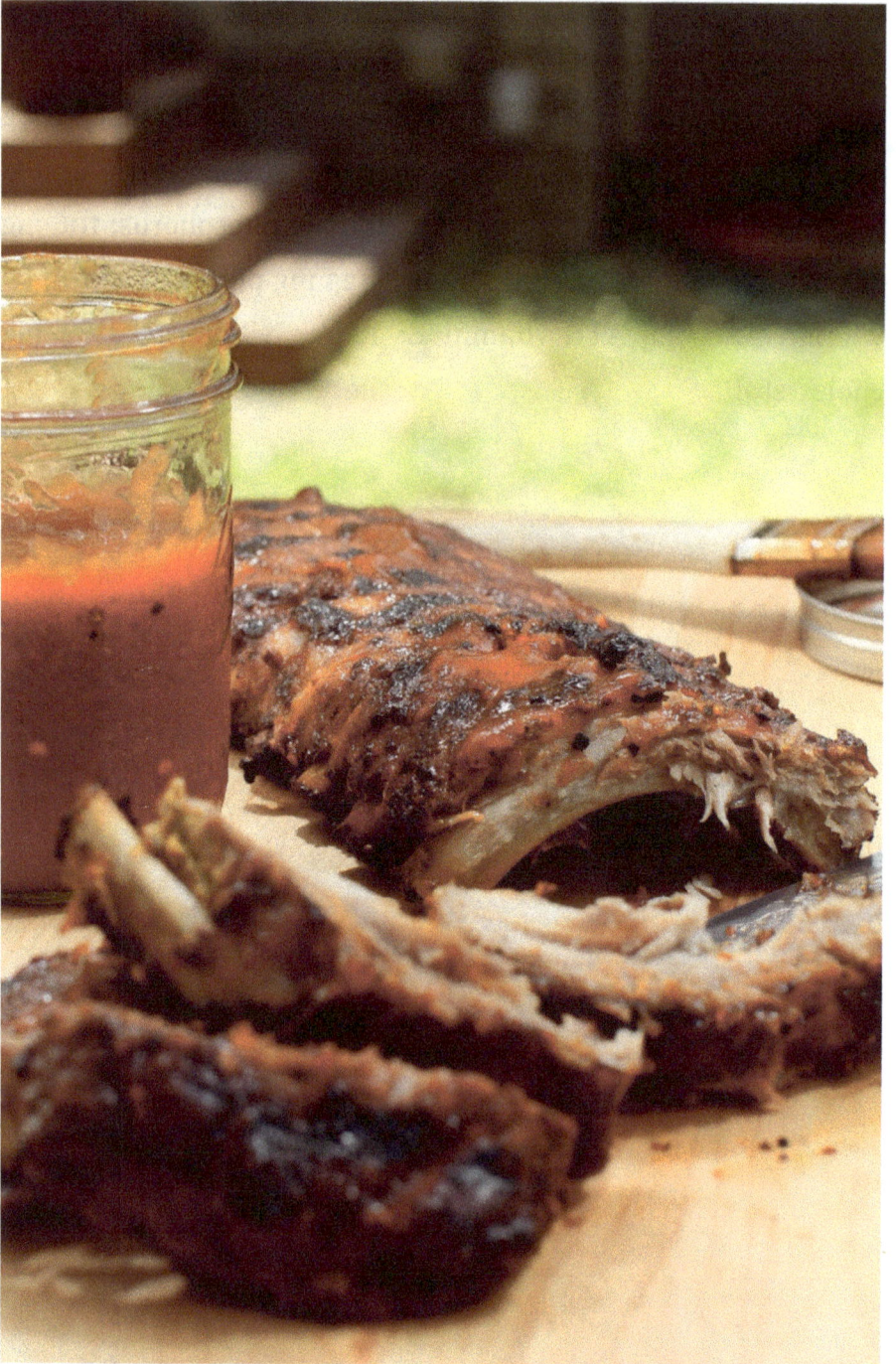

Ham And Scalloped Potatoes

Servings: 8 Servings

Ingredients:

- 8 medium potatoes, peeled and thinly sliced
- ½ teaspoon cream of tartar
- 1 cup (235 ml) water
- 1 pound (455 g) ham, sliced
- 2 cups (320 g) thinly sliced onions
- 1 cup (120 g) grated Cheddar cheese
- 10 ounces (280 g) low-sodium cream of mushroom soup
- Paprika

Directions:

1. Toss sliced potatoes in cream of tartar and water. Drain. Put half of ham, potatoes, and onions in slow cooker. Sprinkle with grated cheese. Repeat with remaining half of ham, potatoes, and onions. Spoon undiluted soup over top. Sprinkle with paprika. Cover and cook on low 8 to 10 hours or on high 4 hours.

Nutrition Info:

Per serving: 378 g water; 435 calories (22% from fat, 21% from protein, 57% from carb); 23 g protein; 11 g total fat; 5 g saturated fat; 4 g monounsaturated fat; 1 g polyunsaturated fat; 63 g carb; 7 g fiber; 5 g sugar; 446 mg phosphorus; 169 mg calcium; 3 mg iron; 732 mg sodium; 1953 mg potassium; 192 IU vitamin A; 43 mg ATE vitamin E; 35 mg vitamin C; 41 mg cholesterol

Pork And Pineapple Roast

Servings: About 4

Cooking Time: 7 Hrs

Ingredients:

- 2 pounds Pork Roast
- 1.5 tsp. Salt
- ½ tsp. Black Pepper
- 20-ounces Pineapple Chunks
-
- 1 cup Cranberries (chopped)

Directions:

1. Season the roast on all sides.
2. Place all the ingredients in the slow cooker.
3. Cook on "low" for 7 hrs.
4. Serve hot.

Nutrition Info:

(Estimated Amount Per Serving): 465.1 Calories; 10.7 g Total Fat; 134.3 mg Cholesterol; 107.2 mg Sodium; 44.3 mg Carbohydrates; 3 g Dietary Fiber; 47.49 g Protein

Barbecued Brisket

Servings: 10 Servings

Ingredients:

- 4 pounds (1.8 kg) beef brisket
- 12 ounces (355 ml) beer
- 1 can (8 ounces, or 225 g) no-salt-added tomato sauce
- 2 teaspoons prepared mustard
- 2 tablespoons (28 ml) balsamic vinegar
- 2 tablespoons (28 ml) Worcestershire sauce
- 1 teaspoon garlic powder
- ½ teaspoon ground allspice
- 1 tablespoon (15 g) brown sugar
- 1 cup (150 g) chopped red bell pepper
- 1 cup (160 g) chopped onion
- ¼ teaspoon pepper

Directions:

1. Place brisket in slow cooker. Combine remaining ingredients. Pour over meat. Cover and cook on low 8 to 10 hours. Remove meat from sauce. Slice very thinly.

Nutrition Info:

Per serving: 217 g water; 274 calories (25% from fat, 63% from protein, 12% from carb); 40 g protein; 7 g total fat; 3 g saturated fat; 3 g monounsaturated fat; 0 g polyunsaturated fat; 8 g carb; 1 g fiber; 4 g sugar; 392 mg phosphorus; 41 mg calcium; 4 mg iron; 170 mg sodium; 795 mg potassium; 552 IU vitamin A; 0 mg ATE vitamin E; 29 mg vitamin C; 74 mg cholesterol

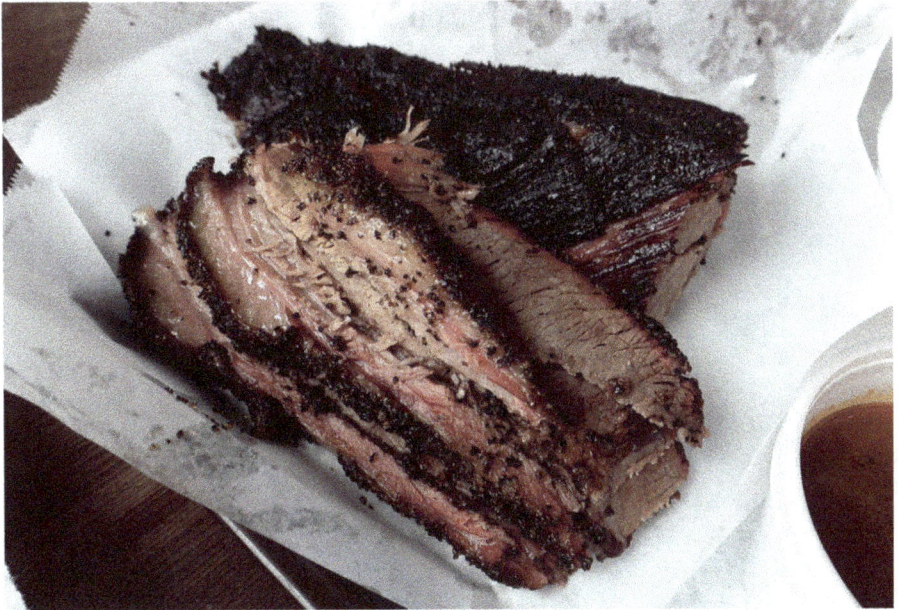

Barbecued Short Ribs

Servings: 10 Servings

Ingredients:

- 2/3 cup (83 g) flour
- ½ teaspoon pepper
- 4 pounds (1.8 kg) beef short ribs
- ¼ cup (60 ml) olive oil
- 1 cup (160 g) chopped onion
- 1½ cups (355 ml) low-sodium beef broth
- ¾ cup (175 ml) red wine vinegar
- ¾ cup (170 g) packed brown sugar
- ½ cup (140 g) chili sauce
- 1/3 cup (80 g) low-sodium ketchup
- 1/3 cup (80 ml) Worcestershire sauce
- 1½ teaspoons minced garlic
- 1½ teaspoons chili powder

Directions:

1. In a large resealable plastic bag, combine the flour and pepper. Add ribs in batches and shake to coat. In a large skillet, heat the oil over medium-high heat and brown ribs on both sides. Transfer to a slow

cooker. In the same skillet, combine the remaining ingredients. Cook and stir until mixture comes to a boil; pour over ribs. Cover and cook on low for 9 to 10 hours or until meat is tender.

Nutrition Info:

Per serving: 213 g water; 488 calories (45% from fat, 31% from protein, 24% from carb); 37 g protein; 24 g total fat; 9 g saturated fat; 12 g monounsaturated fat; 1 g polyunsaturated fat; 29 g carb; 1 g fiber; 19 g sugar; 381 mg phosphorus; 43 mg calcium; 5 mg iron; 241 mg sodium; 867 mg potassium; 400 IU vitamin A; 0 mg ATE vitamin E; 20 mg vitamin C; 107 mg cholesterol

Beer-braised Short Ribs

Servings: 8 Servings

Ingredients:

- 3 pounds (1/3 kg) beef short ribs
- 2 tablespoons (30 g) packed brown sugar
- 1 teaspoon minced garlic
- ¼ cup (31 g) flour
- 1 cup (160 g) chopped onion
- 1 cup (235 ml) low-sodium beef broth
- 12 ounces (355 ml) beer, preferably ale or dark beer

Directions:

1. Place the beef in the slow cooker. Add the brown sugar, garlic, and flour. Toss to coat. Place onions over top. Stir the broth and beer in a small bowl. Pour over the beef. Cover and cook on low for 8 to 9 hours or until the beef is fork-tender.

Nutrition Info:

Per serving: 205 g water; 350 calories (47% from fat, 41% from protein, 12% from carb); 34 g protein; 17 g total fat; 7 g saturated fat; 7 g monounsaturated fat; 1 g polyunsaturated fat; 10 g carb;

0 g fiber; 4 g sugar; 344 mg phosphorus; 26 mg calcium; 4 mg iron; 132 mg sodium; 682 mg potassium; 0 IU vitamin A; 0 mg ATE vitamin E; 2 mg vitamin C; 100 mg cholesterol

Pork And Sweet Potato Dinner

Servings: 6 Servings

Ingredients:

- 3 pounds (1 1/3 kg) boneless pork loin roast
- 4 sweet potatoes, peeled
- 2 medium apples, sliced
- ¼ cup (60 ml) apple juice or white wine
- 2 tablespoons (30 g) brown sugar
- ½ teaspoon apple pie spice

Directions:

1. Cube the pork and the sweet potatoes into bite-size pieces. In a skillet, brown the pork cubes. In the bottom of the slow cooker place apple slices, then sweet potatoes, then browned pork cubes. Combine juice, brown sugar, and apple pie spice and pour over the pork. Cook on low for 8 to 12 hours.

Nutrition Info:

Per serving: 290 g water; 464 calories (30% from fat, 45% from protein, 25% from carb); 51 g protein; 15 g total fat; 5 g saturated fat; 7 g monounsaturated fat; 2 g polyunsaturated fat; 29 g carb;

3 g fiber; 16 g sugar; 508 mg phosphorus; 45 mg calcium; 3 mg iron; 132 mg sodium; 1253 mg potassium; 15877 IU vitamin A; 5 mg ATE vitamin E; 15 mg vitamin C; 125 mg cholesterol

Lamb Stew

Ingredients:

- 2 pounds (900 g) lean lamb
- 2 tablespoons (28 ml) olive oil
- 1 onion, cut in wedges
- ½ teaspoon minced garlic
- 10 ounces (280 g) low-sodium cream of mushroom soup
- ½ cup (120 ml) water
- ½ teaspoon thyme
- 8 ounces (225 g) fat-free sour cream
- 2 tablespoons (16 g) flour

Directions:

1. Cut lamb in 1-inch (2.5 cm) cubes. Heat oil in a large skillet over medium-high heat and brown meat. Transfer to a slow cooker. Add onion and garlic to skillet; cook until onion is tender but not brown. Stir in soup, water, and thyme, scraping browned bits from bottom of skillet. Pour over lamb in slow cooker. Cover and cook on low for 8 to 10 hours. Turn cooker to high. Thoroughly blend sour cream and

flour. Slowly stir 1 cup (235 ml) hot liquid from the slow cooker into the sour cream mixture; return mixture to hot stew. Cover and cook until thickened, 15 minutes.

Nutrition Info:

Per serving: 211 g water; 417 calories (46% from fat, 44% from protein, 10% from carb); 45 g protein; 21 g total fat; 8 g saturated fat; 9 g monounsaturated fat; 2 g polyunsaturated fat; 10 g carb; 1 g fiber; 2 g sugar; 410 mg phosphorus; 74 mg calcium; 4 mg iron; 313 mg sodium; 776 mg potassium; 148 IU vitamin A; 39 mg ATE vitamin E; 2 mg vitamin C; 152 mg cholesterol

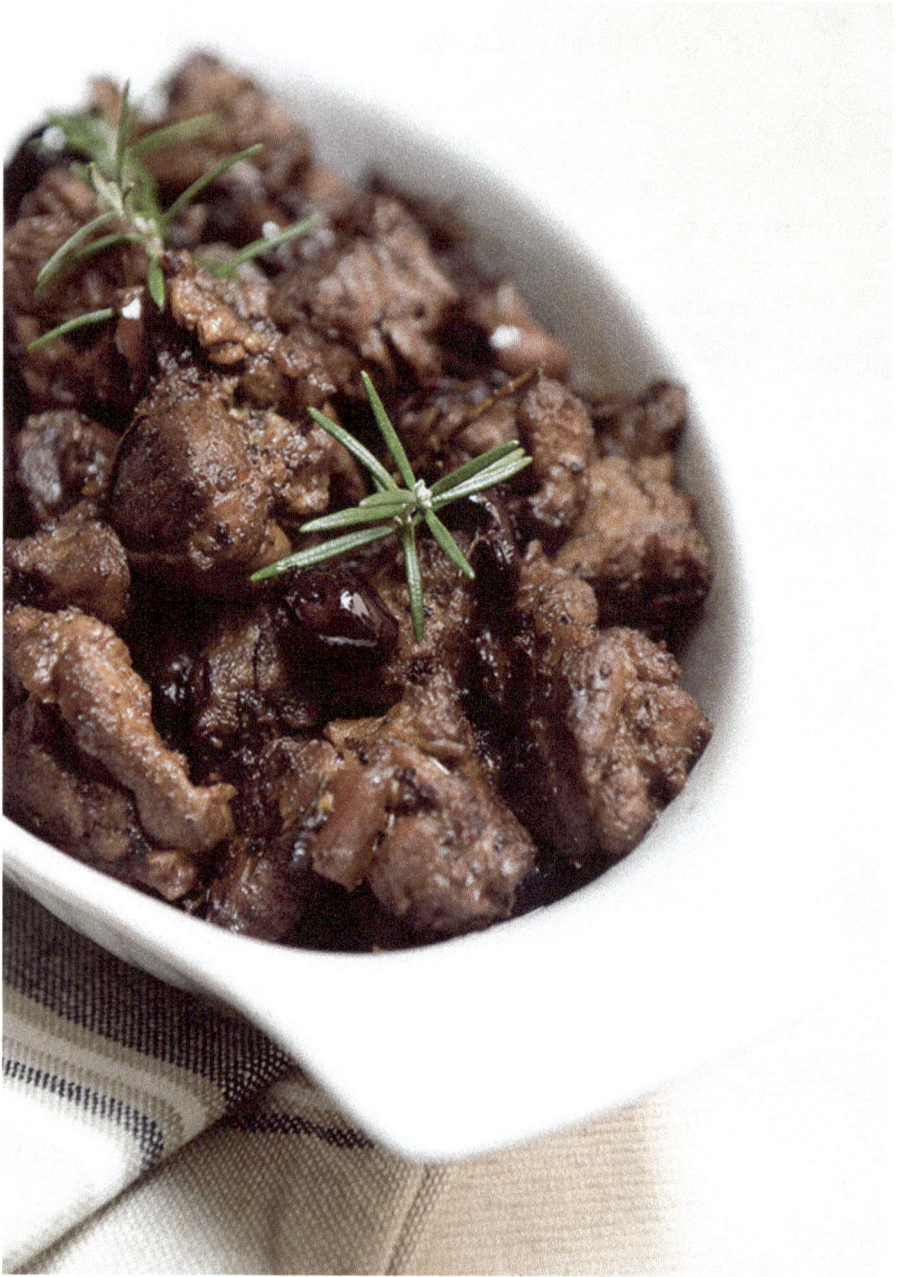

Barbecued Ham

Servings: 24 Servings

Ingredients:

- 2 cups (360 g) sliced onions
- 6 whole cloves
- 3 pounds (1 1/3 kg) reduced-sodium boneless ham
- 2 cups (475 ml) water 2 cups (500 g) barbecue sauce

Directions:

1. Place half of the onions in bottom of slow cooker. Stick cloves in ham and place it on top of onions in slow cooker. Put the rest of the onions on top. Add water. Cook on low 10 to 12 hours. Shred or cut up meat and onion. Put back into slow cooker. Add barbecue sauce. Cook 4 to 6 hours more.

Nutrition Info:

Per serving: 83 g water; 101 calories (15% from fat, 41% from protein, 43% from carb); 10 g protein; 2 g total fat; 1 g saturated fat; 1 g monounsaturated fat; 0 g polyunsaturated fat; 11 g carb; 0 g fiber; 7 g sugar; 127 mg phosphorus; 9 mg calcium; 0 mg

iron; 587 mg sodium; 218 mg potassium; 0 IU vitamin A; 0 mg ATE vitamin E; 1 mg vitamin C; 27 mg cholesterol

Barbecued Beef Roast

Servings: 8 Servings

Ingredients:

- 4 pounds (1.8 kg) beef round roast
- 1 cup (240 g) low-sodium ketchup
- 1 cup (160 g) chopped onion
- ¾ cup (175 ml) water
- ¼ cup (60 ml) Worcestershire sauce
- ¾ cup (170 g) brown sugar

Directions:

1. Place roast in slow cooker. Combine remaining ingredients and pour over. Cover and cook on low for 6 to 10 hours.

Nutrition Info:

Per serving: 229 g water; 411 calories (19% from fat, 51% from protein, 31% from carb); 51 g protein; 8 g total fat; 3 g saturated fat; 4 g monounsaturated fat; 0 g polyunsaturated fat; 31 g carb; 0 g fiber; 28 g sugar; 520 mg phosphorus; 76 mg calcium; 5 mg iron; 230 mg sodium; 1094 mg potassium; 288 IU vitamin A; 0 mg ATE vitamin E; 20 mg vitamin C; 113 mg cholesterol

Lemony Pork Roast

Servings: About 8

Cooking Time: 8 Hrs 15 Mins

Ingredients:

- 4 boneless Pork Chops
- Ground Black Pepper
- 1 sliced Onion
- 2 tsp. Olive Oil
- 1 minced clove Garlic
- 1 sliced Red Bell Pepper
- ½ tsp. ground Cumin
- ½ tsp. ground Cinnamon
- ½ cup Chicken Broth
- ½ cup Coconut Milk
- 1 diced tart Apple
- 1 cup cubed Squash
- 2 tbsp. chopped Parsley

Directions:

1. Place all ingredients except Pork Chops in the slow cooker.
2. Put the pork chops in afterwards.

3. Cook on "low" for 8 hrs.

4. When cooked, transfer the pork to a cutting board.

5. Leave it for 10 mins and then slice.

6. Transfer the pork and vegetables to heated plates and serve.

Nutrition Info:

(Estimated Amount Per Serving): 317 Calories; 15 g Total Fat; 106 mg Cholesterol; 174 mg Sodium; 12 mg Carbohydrates; 5 g Dietary Fiber; 49 g Protein

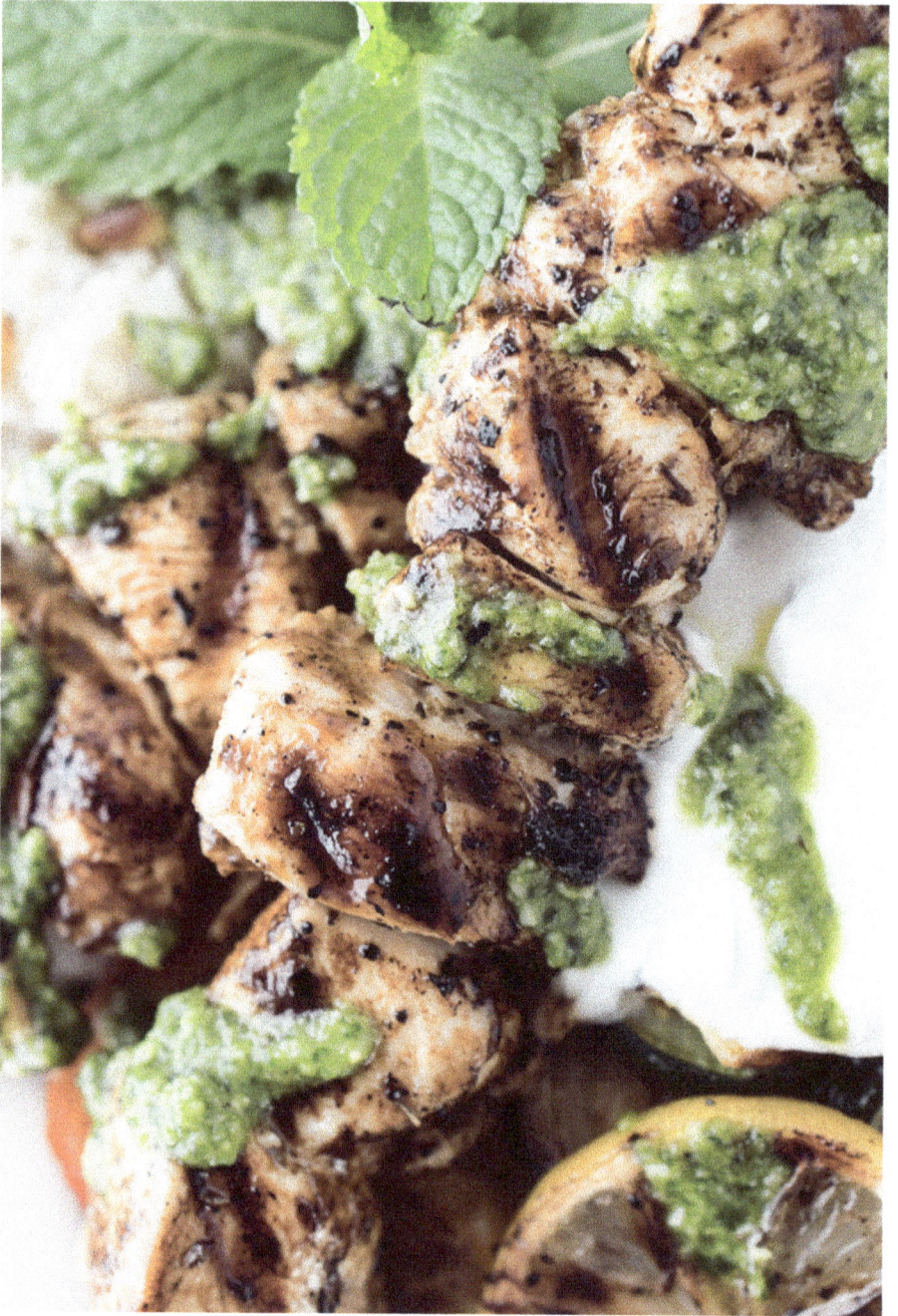

North Carolina Pork

Servings: 15 Servings

Ingredients:

- 5 pounds (2.3 kg) pork shoulder roast
- 1 teaspoon black pepper
- 1½ cups (355 ml) cider vinegar
- 2 tablespoons (30 g) brown sugar
- 1½ tablespoons (23 ml) hot pepper sauce
- 1 teaspoon cayenne

Directions:

1. Place the pork shoulder into a slow cooker and season with pepper. Pour the vinegar around the pork. Cover and cook on low for 12 hours. Pork should easily pull apart into strands. Remove the pork from the slow cooker and discard any bones. Strain out the liquid and save 2 cups (475 ml). Discard any extra. Shred the pork using tongs or two forks and return to the slow cooker. Stir the brown sugar, hot pepper sauce, and cayenne into the reserved liquid. Mix into the pork in the slow cooker. Cover and cook on low for 1 hour more.

Nutrition Info:

Per serving: 121 g water; 370 calories (68% from fat, 29% from protein, 2% from carb); 26 g protein; 27 g total fat; 9 g saturated fat; 12 g monounsaturated fat; 3 g polyunsaturated fat; 2 g carb; 0 g fiber; 2 g sugar; 278 mg phosphorus; 27 mg calcium; 2 mg iron; 109 mg sodium; 486 mg potassium; 83 IU vitamin A; 3 mg ATE vitamin E; 1 mg vitamin C; 107 mg cholesterol

Honey Barbecue Chops

Servings: 8 Servings

Ingredients:

- 8 pork chops
- 1 cup (160 g) sliced onion
- 1 cup (235 ml) low-sodium barbecue sauce
- ¼ cup (85 g) honey

Directions:

1. Place one layer of pork chops in slow cooker. Arrange a proportionate amount of sliced onions over top. Mix barbecue sauce and honey together in a small bowl. Spoon a proportionate amount of sauce over the chops. Repeat the layers with remaining chops, onions, and sauce. Cover and cook on low 6 to 8 hours.

Nutrition Info:

Per serving: 39 g water; 335 cal (40% from fat, 29% from protein, 31% from carb); 24 g protein; 15 g total fat; 5 g saturated fat; 7 g monounsaturated fat; 2 g polyunsaturated fat; 26 g carb; 0 g fiber; 21 g sugar; 6 mg phosphorus; 26 mg calcium; 1 mg iron; 31 mg sodium; 451 mg potassium; 9 IU vitamin A; 0 mg ATE vitamin E; 2 mg vitamin C; 74 mg cholesterol

Beef With Gravy

Servings: 3 Servings

Ingredients:

- 10 ounces (280 g) low-sodium cream of mushroom soup
- 2 tablespoons (28 g) low-sodium onion soup mix
- 1 pound (455 g) beef round steak, cut into 1-inch (2.5 cm) cubes

Directions:

1. Spray the interior of the cooker with nonstick cooking spray. In the slow cooker, combine soup and soup mix. Stir in beef. Cover and cook on low 6 to 8 hours or until meat is tender but not dry.

Nutrition Info:

Per serving: 190 g water; 241 calories (26% from fat, 61% from protein, 13% from carb); 36 g protein; 7 g total fat; 2 g saturated fat; 2 g monounsaturated fat; 1 g polyunsaturated fat; 8 g carb; 1 g fiber; 2 g sugar; 379 mg phosphorus; 17 mg calcium; 4 mg iron; 109 mg sodium; 933 mg potassium; 8 IU vitamin A; 2 mg ATE vitamin E; 0 mg vitamin C; 89 mg cholesterol

Pork Chops with Sweet Potatoes

Servings: 4 Servings

Ingredients:

- 4 pork loin chops
- 1 tablespoon (15 ml) olive oil
- 1 cup (160 g) sliced onions
- 2 sweet potatoes, peeled and cut into large chunks
- 1 cup (235 ml) low-sodium chicken broth

Directions:

1. In a large skillet, heat oil over medium-high heat. Brown pork chops on both sides. Spray the inside surface of a slow cooker with nonstick cooking spray. Arrange sliced onions in the bottom and place pork chops on top of onions. Place sweet potatoes on top. Pour broth over everything. Cover and cook on low for 5 to 6 hours

Nutrition Info:

Per serving: 229 g water; 235 calories (31% from fat, 40% from protein, 30% from carb); 23 g protein; 8 g total fat; 2 g saturated fat; 4 g monounsaturated fat; 1 g polyunsaturated fat; 17 g carb;

3 g fiber; 6 g sugar; 263 mg phosphorus; 45 mg calcium; 2 mg iron; 109 mg sodium; 624 mg potassium; 11892 IU vitamin A; 2 mg ATE vitamin E; 14 mg vitamin C; 64 mg cholesterol

Pork Chops with Apples

Servings: 4 Servings

Ingredients:

- 4 pork loin chops
- 1 cup (160 g) sliced onion
- 2 apples, peeled, cored and sliced
- 1 tablespoon (15 g) brown sugar
- ½ teaspoon nutmeg
- ¼ teaspoon freshly ground black pepper

Directions:

1. Heat a skillet over medium-high heat and coat with cooking spray. Quickly brown the pork chops on each side. Set aside. Arrange onion slices, then the apple slices in slow cooker. Sprinkle brown sugar, nutmeg, and pepper over the apples. Place the pork chops on top. Cover and cook on low for 5 to 6 hours.

Nutrition Info:

Per serving: 165 g water; 191 calories (21% from fat, 46% from protein, 33% from carb); 22 g protein; 4 g total fat; 2 g saturated fat; 2 g monounsaturated fat; 0 g polyunsaturated fat; 15 g carb;

2 g fiber; 12 g sugar; 240 mg phosphorus; 30 mg calcium; 1 mg iron; 55 mg sodium; 504 mg potassium; 33 IU vitamin A; 2 mg ATE vitamin E; 6 mg vitamin C; 64 mg cholesterol

Italian Steak

Servings: 6 Servings

Ingredients:

- 1½ pounds (680 g) beef round steak
- ½ teaspoon oregano
- ¼ teaspoon pepper
- 1 cup (160 g) coarsely chopped onion
- 15 ounces (425 g) low-sodium spaghetti sauce

Directions:

1. Cut steak into 6 pieces. In a bowl, mix together oregano and pepper. Sprinkle over both sides of pieces of meat. Place the meat into the slow cooker. Sprinkle with chopped onion. Spoon spaghetti sauce over top, being careful not to disturb the seasoning and onions. Cover and cook on low 5 to 8 hours or until the meat is tender but not overcooked.

Nutrition Info:

Per serving: 158 g water; 232 calories (28% from fat, 48% from protein, 24% from carb); 27 g protein; 7 g total fat; 2 g saturated fat; 4 g monounsaturated fat; 1 g polyunsaturated fat; 14 g carb;

3 g fiber; 9 g sugar; 282 mg phosphorus; 31 mg calcium; 3 mg iron; 81 mg sodium; 747 mg potassium; 446 IU vitamin A; 0 mg ATE vitamin E; 10 mg vitamin C; 65 mg cholesterol

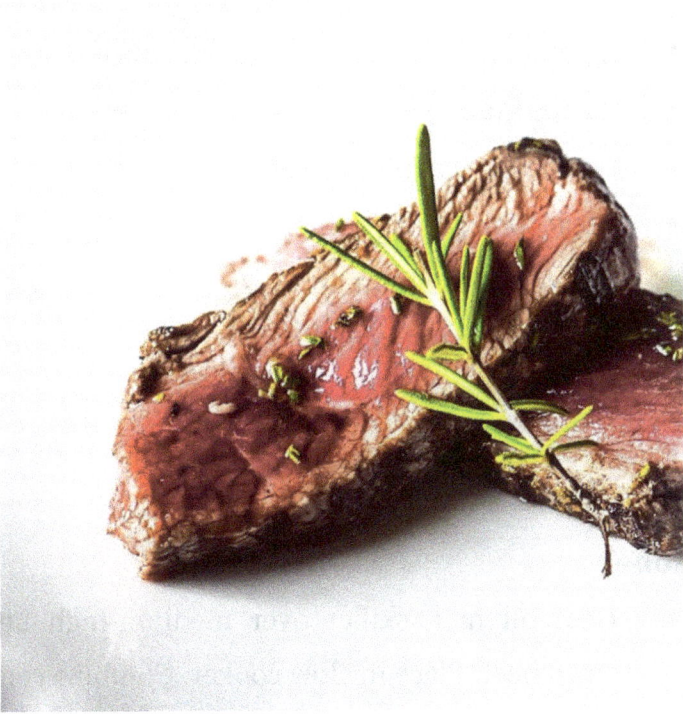

Mexican Brisket

Servings: 8 Servings

Ingredients:

- 2 tablespoons (28 ml) olive oil
- 3 pounds (1 1/3 kg) beef brisket, cubed
- 2 cups (520 g) low-sodium salsa
- 2 tablespoons (28 ml) vinegar
- 1 teaspoon garlic powder
- ½ teaspoon cinnamon
- ½ teaspoon oregano
- ¼ teaspoon cloves
- ¼ teaspoon pepper

Directions:

1. Heat oil in a skillet over medium-high heat and brown beef. Place in slow cooker. Combine remaining ingredients. Pour over meat. Cover and cook on low 10 to 12 hours. Add water as needed.

Nutrition Info:

Per serving: 187 g water; 266 calories (35% from fat, 58% from protein, 7% from carb); 38 g protein; 10 g total fat; 3 g saturated fat; 4 g monounsaturated fat; 2 g polyunsaturated fat; 5 g carb; 1 g fiber; 2 g sugar; 366 mg phosphorus; 48 mg calcium; 4 mg iron; 276 mg sodium; 773 mg potassium; 197 IU vitamin A; 0 mg ATE vitamin E; 2 mg vitamin C; 70 mg cholesterol

Mexican Steak

Servings: 6 Serving s

Ingredients:

- 2 pounds (900 g) flank steak
- ¼ teaspoon garlic powder
- 2 cups (520 g) low-sodium salsa
- 1 can (8 ounces, or 225 g) no-salt-added tomato sauce
- Dash hot pepper sauce
- Monterey Jack cheese, shredded

Directions:

1. Pound meat on both sides with meat mallet; sprinkle with garlic powder. Place in slow cooker. Combine salsa, tomato sauce, and hot pepper sauce. Pour over meat. Cover; cook on low-heat setting for 8 to 10 hours. Sprinkle with cheese before serving.

Nutrition Info:

Per serving: 194 g water; 327 calories (36% from fat, 55% from protein, 9% from carb); 44 g protein; 13 g total fat; 5 g saturated fat; 5 g monounsaturated fat; 1 g polyunsaturated fat; 7 g carb; 2

g fiber; 4 g sugar; 354 mg phosphorus; 47 mg calcium; 3 mg iron; 253 mg sodium; 863 mg potassium; 338 IU vitamin A; 0 mg ATE vitamin E; 6 mg vitamin C; 83 mg cholesterol

Asian Pork Roast

Servings: 8 Servings

Ingredients:

- 3 pounds (1 1/3 kg) pork loin roast
- ½ cup (120 ml) low-sodium soy sauce
- ½ cup (120 ml) sherry
- ½ teaspoon minced garlic
- 1 tablespoon (9 g) dry mustard
- 1 teaspoon ground ginger
- 1 teaspoon thyme

Directions:

1. Place the pork roast in a resealable plastic bag; set in a deep bowl. Thoroughly blend together the soy sauce, sherry, garlic, mustard, ginger, and thyme. Pour marinade over meat in bag; close bag. Place the roast in the refrigerator and marinate for 2 to 3 hours or overnight. Transfer the pork roast and marinade to a slow cooker. Cover and cook on high for 3½ to 4 hours. Lift roast out onto a cutting board; let stand for 10 minutes before slicing.

Nutrition Info:

Per serving: 147 g water; 253 calories (29% from fat, 65% from protein, 7% from carb); 37 g protein; 7 g total fat; 2 g saturated fat; 3 g monounsaturated fat; 1 g polyunsaturated fat; 4 g carb; 0 g fiber; 1 g sugar; 391 mg phosphorus; 30 mg calcium; 2 mg iron; 138 mg sodium; 680 mg potassium; 18 IU vitamin A; 3 mg ATE vitamin E; 2 mg vitamin C; 107 mg cholesterol

Spanish Steak

Servings: 4 Servings

Ingredients:

- 1 cup (160 g) sliced onion
- ½ cup (50 g) chopped celery
- ¾ cup (113 g) green bell pepper, sliced in rings
- 1 pound (455 g) beef round steak
- 2 teaspoons dried parsley
- 1 tablespoon (15 ml) Worcestershire sauce
- 1 tablespoon (9 g) dry mustard
- 1 tablespoon (7.5 g) chili powder
- 1 cup (180 g) no-salt-added diced tomatoes
- 2 teaspoons minced garlic
- ¼ teaspoon pepper

Directions:

1. Put half of onion, celery, and green pepper in slow cooker. Cut steak into serving-size pieces. Place steak pieces in slow cooker. Put remaining onion, celery, and green pepper over steak. Combine remaining ingredients. Pour over meat. Cover and cook on low 8 hours.

Nutrition Info:

Per serving: 214 g water; 192 calories (21% from fat, 58% from protein, 21% from carb); 28 g protein; 4 g total fat; 1 g saturated fat; 2 g monounsaturated fat; 0 g polyunsaturated fat; 10 g carb; 3 g fiber; 4 g sugar; 292 mg phosphorus; 50 mg calcium; 4 mg iron; 136 mg sodium; 770 mg potassium; 853 IU vitamin A; 0 mg ATE vitamin E; 41 mg vitamin C; 65 mg cholesterol

Chili Beef Roast

Servings: 8 Servings

Ingredients:

- 3 pounds (1 1/3 kg) beef chuck roast
- 2 tablespoons (16 g) flour
- 1 tablespoon (11 g) prepared mustard
- 1 tablespoon (20 g) chili sauce
- 1 tablespoon (15 ml) Worcestershire sauce
- 1 teaspoon cider vinegar
- 1 tablespoon (7.5 g) chili powder
- 1 teaspoon sugar
- 4 potatoes, sliced
- 1 cup (160 g) sliced onions

Directions:

1. Place roast in slow cooker. Make a paste with the flour, mustard, chili sauce, Worcestershire sauce, vinegar, chili powder, and sugar. Spread over the roast. Top with potatoes and then the onions. Cover and cook on low 10 to 12 hours.

Nutrition Info:

Per serving: 270 g water; 511 calories (24% from fat, 48% from protein, 27% from carb); 60 g protein; 13 g total fat; 5 g saturated fat; 5 g monounsaturated fat; 1 g polyunsaturated fat; 34 g carb; 4 g fiber; 3 g sugar; 581 mg phosphorus; 43 mg calcium; 8 mg iron; 154 mg sodium; 1399 mg potassium; 326 IU vitamin A; 0 mg ATE vitamin E; 22 mg vitamin C; 172 mg cholesterol

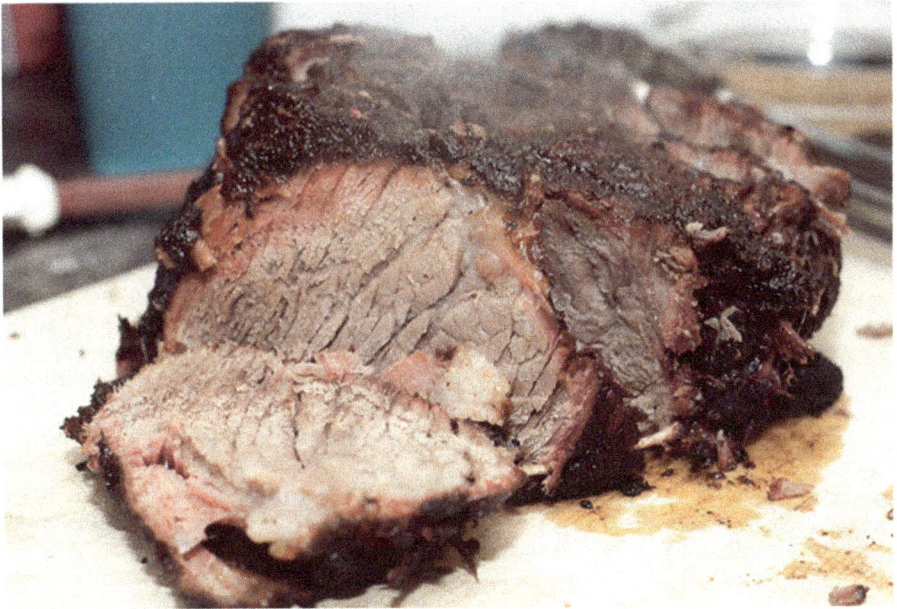

Pork Chops with Mushrooms

Servings: 6 Servings

Ingredients:

- 10 ounces (280 g) low-sodium cream of mushroom soup
- 1 cup (160 g) chopped onion
- 8 ounces (225 g) mushrooms, sliced
- 1 teaspoon Worcestershire sauce
- 6 boneless pork loin chops

Directions:

1. Mix soup, onions, and mushrooms. Stir in Worcestershire sauce. Pour half of mixture into slow cooker. Place pork chops in slow cooker. Cover with the remaining sauce. Cover and cook on low 4 to 5 hours or until meat is tender but not dry.

Nutrition Info:

Per serving: 174 g water; 173 calories (27% from fat, 55% from protein, 18% from carb); 23 g protein; 5 g total fat; 2 g saturated fat; 2 g monounsaturated fat; 1 g polyunsaturated fat; 8 g carb; 1 g fiber; 3 g sugar; 285 mg phosphorus; 27 mg calcium; 1 mg

iron; 78 mg sodium; 716 mg potassium; 12 IU vitamin A; 3 mg ATE vitamin E; 5 mg vitamin C; 65 mg cholesterol

Brisket with Mixed Potatoes

Servings: 8 Servings

Ingredients:

- 3 large potatoes, peeled and cut into 1-inch (2.5 cm) cubes
- 3 sweet potatoes, peeled and cut into 1-inch (2.5 cm) cubes
- 3 pounds (1 1/3 kg) beef brisket, fat trimmed
- 1 cup (260 g) low-sodium salsa

Directions:

1. Place both kinds of potatoes in the slow cooker. Top with the brisket. Pour salsa evenly over the meat. Cover and cook either on low 8 to 10 hours or on high 4 to 5 hours until the meat is tender but not dry. To serve, remove the meat from the cooker, keep warm, and allow to rest for 10 minutes. Then slice the meat across the grain. Place slices on a platter and top with the potatoes and sauce.

Nutrition Info:

Per serving: 312 g water; 365 calories (17% from fat, 45% from protein, 38% from carb); 41 g protein; 7 g total fat; 2 g saturated fat; 3 g monounsaturated fat; 0 g polyunsaturated fat; 34 g carb; 4 g fiber; 6 g sugar; 456 mg phosphorus; 65 mg calcium; 5 mg iron; 224 mg sodium; 1428 mg potassium; 9017 IU vitamin A; 0 mg ATE vitamin E; 20 mg vitamin C; 70 mg cholesterol

Italian Beef Roast

Servings: 10 Servings

Ingredients:

- 2½ cups (570 ml) water
- 2 tablespoons (28 g) onion soup mix
- 2 tablespoons (28 ml) Worcestershire sauce
- 1 teaspoon garlic powder
- 1 teaspoon marjoram
- 1 teaspoon thyme
- 1 teaspoon oregano
- 4 pounds (1.8 kg) beef chuck roast

Directions:

1. In a slow cooker, combine the water, soup mix, Worcestershire sauce, garlic powder, marjoram, thyme, and oregano. Add the meat. Cook for either 4 to 6 hours on high or 8 to 10 hours on low until the meat falls apart. Pull the meat apart and use for sandwiches or over pasta.

Nutrition Info:

Per serving: 166 g water; 385 calories (34% from fat, 65% from protein, 1% from carb); 60 g protein; 14 g total fat; 5 g saturated fat; 6 g monounsaturated fat; 1 g polyunsaturated fat; 1 g carb; 0 g fiber; 0 g sugar; 491 mg phosphorus; 23 mg calcium; 7 mg iron; 151 mg sodium; 555 mg potassium; 18 IU vitamin A; 0 mg ATE vitamin E; 6 mg vitamin C; 183 mg cholesterol

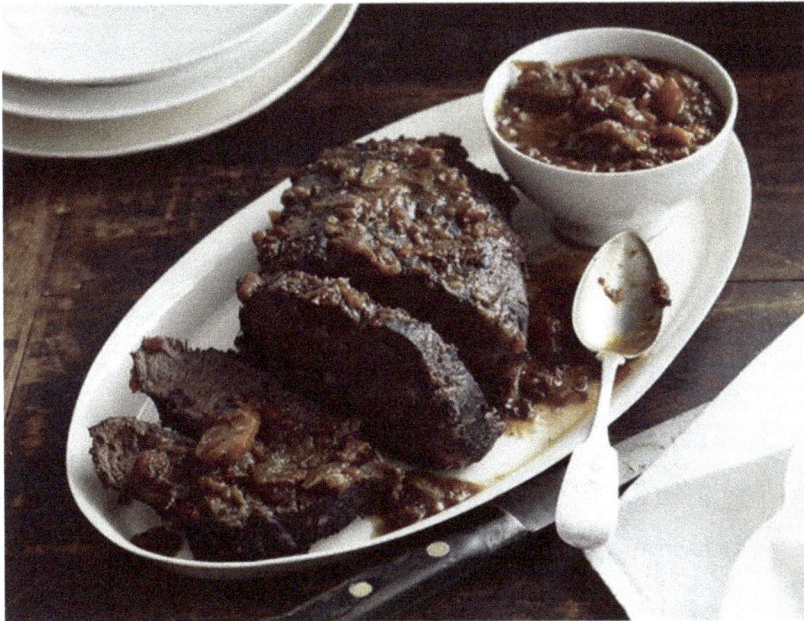

Lamb Paprikash

Servings: 6 Servings

Ingredients:

- 2 pounds (900 g) lamb, cut in 1-inch (2.5 cm) pieces
- 1 can (14 ounces, or 400 g) no-salt-added diced tomatoes
- 1 cup (160 g) chopped onion
- ½ teaspoon minced garlic
- 1 teaspoon paprika
- ½ cup (120 ml) cold water
- ¼ cup (31 g) flour
- ½ cup (115 g) fat-free sour cream

Directions:

1. In slow cooker, combine lamb, undrained tomatoes, onion, garlic, and paprika. Cover and cook on low for 8 to 10 hours. Turn cooker to high; spoon off any excess fat. Blend cold water slowly into flour; stir into the meat mixture. Cover and cook until thickened and bubbly, 20 to 30 minutes. Blend about ½ cup (120 ml) of the hot liquid from the slow cooker into the sour cream; stir sour cream mixture into cooker. Heat through.

Nutrition Info:

Per serving: 219 g water; 351 calories (36% from fat, 52% from protein, 12% from carb); 44 g protein; 14 g total fat; 6 g saturated fat; 5 g monounsaturated fat; 1 g polyunsaturated fat; 10 g carb; 1 g fiber; 3 g sugar; 385 mg phosphorus; 70 mg calcium; 5 mg iron; 134 mg sodium; 712 mg potassium; 355 IU vitamin A; 20 mg ATE vitamin E; 9 mg vitamin C; 144 mg cholesterol

Marinated Pot Roast

Servings: 6 Servings

Ingredients:

- 3 pounds (1 1/3 kg) beef chuck roast
- 1½ cups (355 ml) low-sodium tomato juice
- ¼ cup (60 ml) red wine vinegar
- ½ teaspoon minced garlic
- 2 teaspoons Worcestershire sauce
- ½ teaspoon basil
- ½ teaspoon thyme
- ¼ teaspoon pepper
- 1 cup (160 g) chopped onion
- 1 cup (130 g) sliced carrot
- ½ cup (120 ml) cold water
- ¼ cup (31 g) flour

Directions:

1. Trim excess fat from roast. If necessary, cut roast in halves or thirds to fit in cooker. Place meat in a resealable plastic bag; set in deep bowl. Stir together tomato juice, vinegar, garlic, Worcestershire sauce, basil, thyme, and pepper. Pour marinade over meat;

close bag. Marinate overnight in refrigerator, turning twice. Place onions and carrot In slow cooker. Place roast on top of vegetables; add marinade. Cover and cook on low for 8 to 10 hours. Remove roast and vegetables. Skim off excess fat from cooking liquid. Measure 2 cups (475 ml) cooking liquid; pour into saucepan. Return meat and vegetables to cooker; cover to keep warm. Blend cold water slowly into flour; stir into reserved cooking liquid in saucepan. Cook and stir until mixture is thickened and bubbly. Place meat on a warm serving platter; top with vegetables. Pour some of the gravy over; pass the remaining gravy at the table.

Nutrition Info:

Per serving: 263 g water; 529 calories (31% from fat, 60% from protein, 9% from carb); 76 g protein; 17 g total fat; 6 g saturated fat; 7 g monounsaturated fat; 1 g polyunsaturated fat; 12 g carb; 1 g fiber; 4 g sugar; 643 mg phosphorus; 45 mg calcium; 9 mg iron; 189 mg sodium; 929 mg potassium; 3875 IU vitamin A; 0 mg ATE vitamin E; 18 mg vitamin C; 229 mg cholesterol

Red Beans

Servings: 6 Servings

Ingredients:

- 1 pound (455 g) dried kidney beans
- ½ teaspoon chopped garlic
- 1 cup (160 g) finely chopped onion
- ½ cup (50 g) chopped celery
- 1 pound (455 g) smoked sausage, browned and cut in thin slices
- 3 bay leaves
- 6 cups (1.4 L) water

Directions:

1. Wash beans and cover with water, boil until done (about 1 hour) and then drain. In a skillet, sauté garlic, onion, and celery. Add to beans after beans are cooked. Add browned sausage and bay leaves. Put all ingredients in slow cooker with 6 cups (4 L) water; cover and cook on low for 2 to 2½ hours. Remove bay leaves before serving.

Nutrition Info:

Per serving: 366 g water; 276 calories (43% from fat, 25% from protein, 32% from carb); 17 g protein; 13 g total fat; 5 g saturated fat; 6 g monounsaturated fat; 2 g polyunsaturated fat; 22 g carb; 8 g fiber; 1 g sugar; 117 mg phosphorus; 50 mg calcium; 3 mg iron; 532 mg sodium; 350 mg potassium; 41 IU vitamin A; 0 mg ATE vitamin E; 14 mg vitamin C; 53 mg cholesterol

German Beef Roast

Servings: 8 Servings

Ingredients:

- 4 pounds (1.8 kg) beef chuck roast
- 1/3 cup (80 ml) cider vinegar
- 1 cup (160 g) sliced onion
- 3 bay leaves
- ¼ teaspoon cloves
- ¼ teaspoon garlic powder
- ½ teaspoon ginger

Directions:

1. Place roast in slow cooker. Add remaining ingredients. Cover and cook on low 8 to 10 hours. Remove bay leaves before serving.

Nutrition Info:

Per serving: 160 g water; 487 calories (33% from fat, 65% from protein, 2% from carb); 75 g protein; 17 g total fat; 6 g saturated fat; 7 g monounsaturated fat; 1 g polyunsaturated fat; 2 g carb; 0 g fiber; 1 g sugar; 615 mg phosphorus; 26 mg calcium; 9 mg

iron; 151 mg sodium; 695 mg potassium; 1 IU vitamin A; 0 mg
ATE vitamin E; 2 mg vitamin C; 229 mg cholesterol

Beef Paprikash

Servings: 8 Servings

Ingredients:

- 2 pounds (900 g) beef round steak, cubed
- 1 cup (160 g) sliced onion
- ½ teaspoon garlic powder
- ½ cup (120 g) low-sodium ketchup
- 2 tablespoons (28 ml) Worcestershire sauce
- 2 tablespoons (30 g) brown sugar
- 2 teaspoons paprika
- ½ teaspoon dry mustard

Directions:

1. Place beef in slow cooker. Cover with onion. Combine remaining ingredients and pour over meat. Cover and cook on low for 8 hours.

Nutrition Info:

Per serving: 110 g water; 185 calories (19% from fat, 58% from protein, 22% from carb); 27 g protein; 4 g total fat; 1 g saturated fat; 1 g monounsaturated fat; 0 g polyunsaturated fat; 10 g carb; 1 g fiber; 8 g sugar; 267 mg phosphorus; 15 mg calcium; 3 mg

iron; 101 mg sodium; 579 mg potassium; 448 IU vitamin A; 0 mg ATE vitamin E; 11 mg vitamin C; 65 mg cholesterol

Greek Sandwich Filling

Servings: 16 Servings

Ingredients:

- 4 tablespoons (60 ml) olive oil, divided
- 4 pounds (1.8 kg) beef round steak, cut in ½-inch (1.3 cm) cubes, divided
- 2 cups (320 g) chopped onions
- ½ teaspoon minced garlic
- 1 cup (235 ml) dry red wine
- 1 can (6 ounces, or 170 g) no-salt-added tomato paste
- 1 teaspoon oregano
- 1 teaspoon basil
- ½ teaspoon rosemary
- Dash black pepper
- 1 tablespoon (8 g) cornstarch
- 2 tablespoons (28 ml) water

Directions:

1. Heat 1 tablespoon (15 ml) oil in a skillet and then add 1 pound (455 g) meat and brown. Repeat with remaining oil and meat. Reserve drippings and

transfer meat to slow cooker. Sauté onion and garlic in drippings until tender. Add to meat. Add wine, tomato paste, oregano, basil, rosemary, salt, and pepper. Cover and cook on low 6 to 8 hours. Turn cooker to high. Combine cornstarch and water in small bowl until smooth. Stir into meat mixture. Cook until bubbly and thickened, stirring occasionally.

Nutrition Info:

Per serving: 119 g water; 204 calories (34% from fat, 56% from protein, 9% from carb); 27 g protein; 7 g total fat; 2 g saturated fat; 4 g monounsaturated fat; 1 g polyunsaturated fat; 4 g carb; 1 g fiber; 2 g sugar; 267 mg phosphorus; 15 mg calcium; 3 mg iron; 71 mg sodium; 593 mg potassium; 171 IU vitamin A; 0 mg ATE vitamin E; 4 mg vitamin C; 65 mg cholesterol

Pork Roast

Servings: About 8

Cooking Time: 10 Hrs

Ingredients:

- 2 lbs Pork Roast (Sirloin)
- 1 envelope Lipton Onion Soup Mix
- 1 can Chicken Soup
- 1 tsp. Thyme (dried)
- 1 tsp. Rosemary (dried)
- ¼ tsp. Red Pepper Flakes
- ½ tsp. ground Black Pepper
- 2 cups Water

Directions:

1. Mix all the ingredients in the slow cooker.
2. Cook on "low" for 10 hrs.
3. Serve hot

Nutrition Info:

(Estimated Amount Per Serving):162.8 Calories; 3.5 g Total Fat; 83.3 mg Cholesterol; 919.9 mg Sodium; 6.1 mg Carbohydrates; 0.5 g Dietary Fiber; 28.8 g Protein

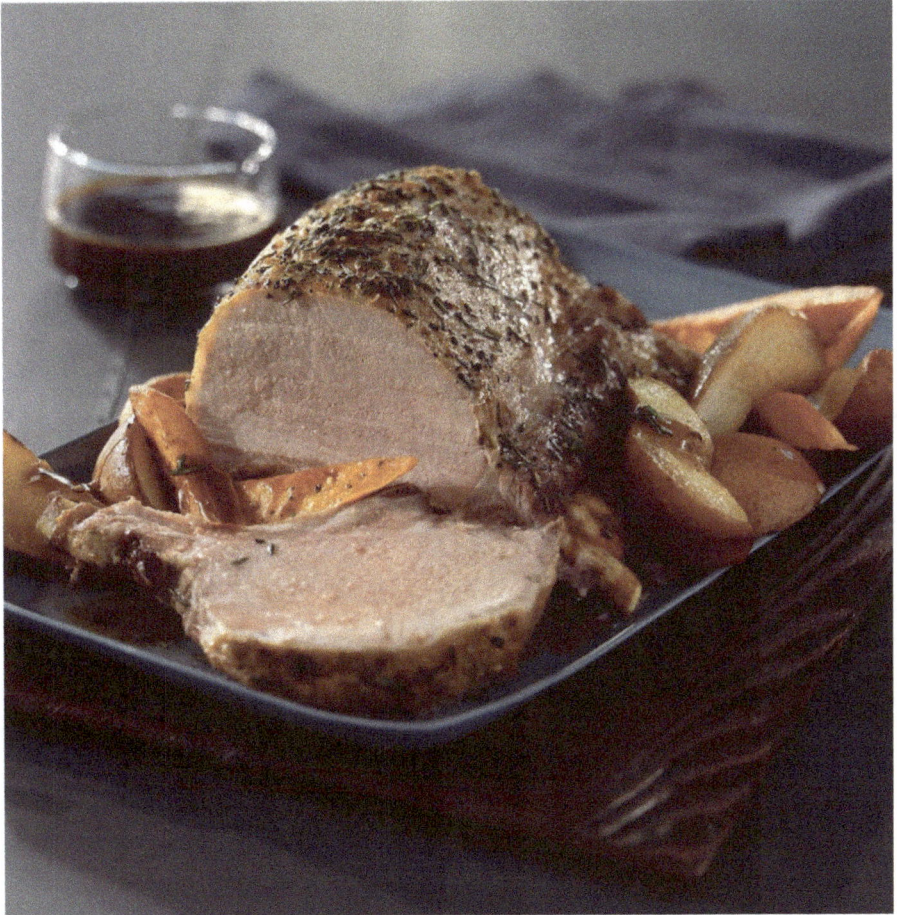

4-WEEK MEAL PLAN

Week 1

Monday
Breakfast: Tofu Frittata
Lunch: Pork Chops In Beer
Dinner: Stewed Tomatoes

Tuesday
Breakfast: Tapioca
Lunch: Creamy Beef Burgundy
Dinner: Oregano Salad

Wednesday
Breakfast: Fruit Oats
Lunch: Smothered Steak
Dinner: Black Beans With Corn Kernels

Thursday
Breakfast: Grapefruit Mix
Lunch: Pork For Sandwiches
Dinner: Stuffed Acorn Squash

Friday
Breakfast: Berry Yogurt
Lunch: Cranberry Pork Roast

Dinner: Greek Eggplant

Saturday
Breakfast: Soft Pudding
Lunch: Pan-asian Pot Roast
Dinner: Thyme Sweet Potatoes

Sunday
Breakfast: Black Beans Salad
Lunch: Short Ribs
Dinner: Barley Vegetable Soup

Week 2

Monday
Breakfast: Carrot Pudding
Lunch: French Dip
Dinner: Butter Corn

Tuesday
Breakfast: Apple Cake
Lunch: Italian Roast With Vegetables
Dinner: Orange Glazed Carrots

Wednesday
Breakfast: Almond Milk Barley Cereals
Lunch: Honey Mustard Ribs
Dinner: Cinnamon Acorn Squash

Thursday

Breakfast: Cashews Cake

Lunch: Pizza Casserole

Dinner: Glazed Root Vegetables

Friday

Breakfast: Artichoke Frittata

Lunch: Hawaiian Pork Roast

Dinner: Stir Fried Steak, Shiitake And Asparagus

Saturday

Breakfast: Mexican Eggs

Lunch: Apple Cranberry Pork Roast

Dinner: Cilantro Brussel Sprouts

Sunday

Breakfast: Stewed Peach

Lunch: Swiss Steak

Dinner: Italian Zucchini

Week 3

Monday

Breakfast: Lamb Cassoule t

Lunch: Glazed Pork Roast

Dinner: Cilantro Parsnip Chunks

Tuesday

Breakfast: Fruited Tapioca

Lunch: Swiss Steak In Wine Sauce

Dinner: Corn Casserole

Wednesday

Breakfast: Baby Spinach Shrimp Salad

Lunch: Italian Pork Chops

Dinner: Pilaf With Bella Mushrooms

Thursday

Breakfast: Coconut And Fruit Cake

Lunch: Italian Pot Roast

Dinner: Italian Style Yellow Squash

Friday

Breakfast: Apple And Squash Bowls

Lunch: Beef With Horseradish Sauce

Dinner: Stevia Peas With Marjoram

Saturday

Breakfast: Slow Cooker Chocolate Cake

Lunch: Oriental Pot Roast

Dinner: Broccoli Rice Casserole

Sunday

Breakfast: Fish Omelet

Lunch: Barbecued Ribs

Dinner: Italians Style Mushroom Mix

Week 4

Monday
Breakfast: Brown Cake
Lunch: Ham And Scalloped Pota toes
Dinner: Broccoli Casserole

Tuesday
Breakfast: Stevia And Walnuts Cut Oats
Lunch: Pork And Pineapple Roast

Wednesday
Breakfast: Walnut And Cinnamon Oatmeal
Lunch: Barbecued Brisket
Dinner: Dinner: Slow Cooker Lasagna

Thursday
Breakfast: Tender Rosemary Sweet Potatoes
Lunch: Barbecued Short Ribs
Dinner: Brussels Sprouts Casserole

Friday
Breakfast: Orange And Maple Syrup Quinoa
Lunch: Beer-braised Short Ribs
Dinner: Pasta And Mushrooms

Saturday
Breakfast: Vanilla And Nutmeg Oatmeal
Lunch: Lamb Stew
Dinner: Onion Cabbage

Sunday

Breakfast: Pecans Cake

Lunch: Barbecued Ham

Dinner: Cheese Broccoli

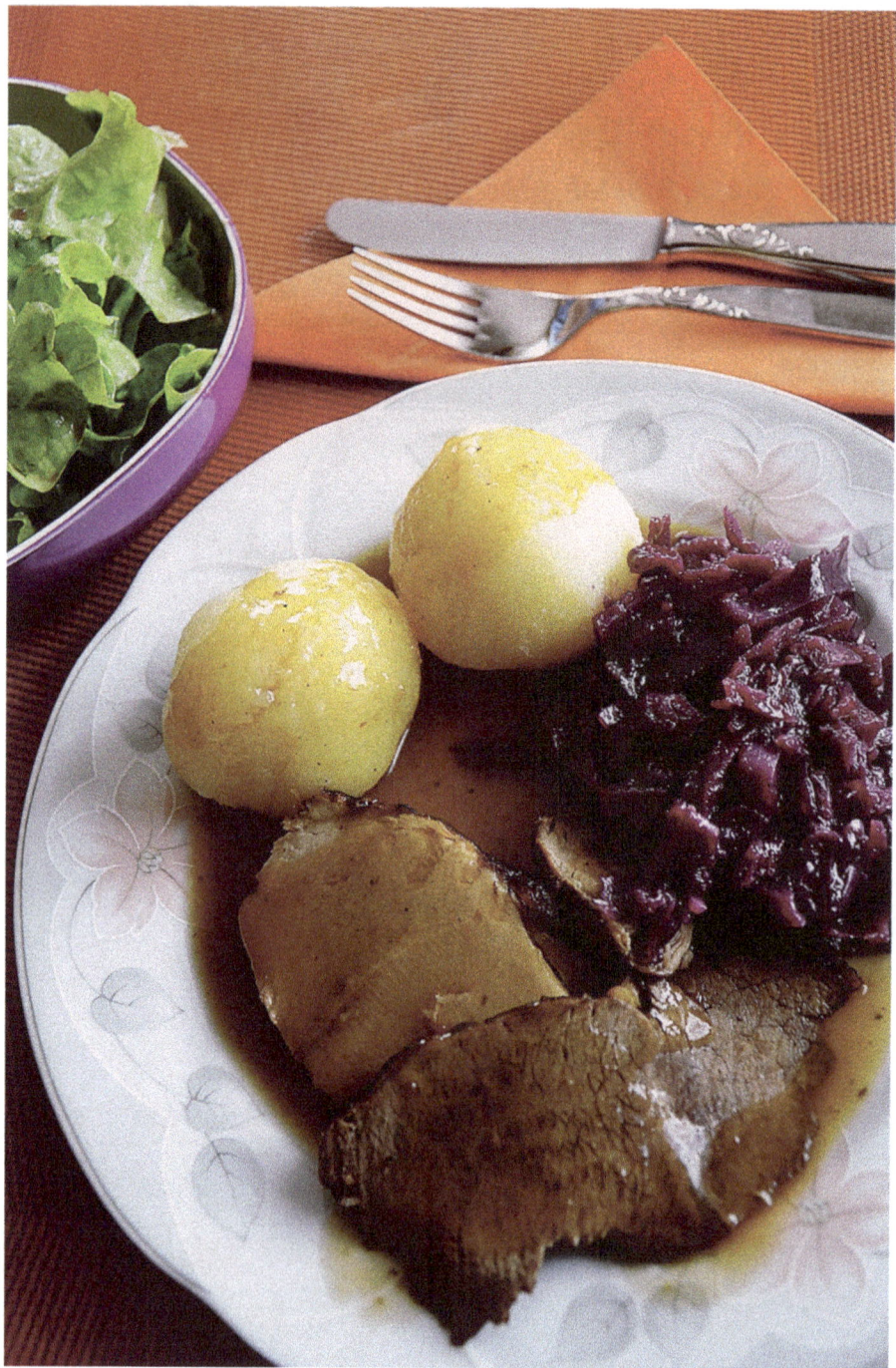

www.ingramcontent.com/pod-product-compliance
Lightning Source LLC
Chambersburg PA
CBHW050217270326
41914CB00003BA/452

a self-afflicted belief that he was intentionally over-looked.

The young woman to whom a man may, possibly, have been introduced by his hostess has the right to allow the acquaintance to go no further than the room in which it occurred, but this is not at all the likely result of a presentation that could not, or would not have been made without the young woman's consent. At the next meeting it is her right, and hers only, to bow a recognition, which, of course, the man acknowledges. If this bow greets him upon the street he can only lift his hat and respond. If it is given to him in society, and the young woman is not occupied by the attentions of another person, he may approach and speak to her ; also with her chaperone's consent ask her to dance with him. If the acquaintance appears to be mutually agreeable, he may ask the chaperone to be allowed the honor of calling at the door to make inquiries after their healths at an early day. She may permit this or she may invite him to call on one of her regular receiving days. More, than this, time develops, or the acquaintance dies for want of interest in one or both.

If he calls, he must ask for her mother, or who-ever is her chaperone first, and then the young woman, placing the elder woman's name first. This is re-spectful courtesy.

When a reception is given for an individual, of course all guests are presented in due form, but phe-

nomenal is the man or woman who is able to remem-
ber and recognize afterwards each individual with
whom speech has been exchanged.

When introductions take place at other than formal
receptions, the man is introduced or presented to the
woman, unless she is young and he old, or distinguished, when she is introduced or presented to him.
Women and men of corresponding ages and social
positions are introduced to each other. Between
equals it is good form to say, " Mrs. B., I should like
you and Mrs. C. to know each other," or, " Permit me
to make two agreeable persons acquainted," or any
other mode of speech is used that does not distinguish
one above the other. The same ceremonial is good
form between men, but between men and women and
between young women and distinguished or elderly
persons, whether men or women, it is good manners to
say to the most important of the two individuals for
example : " Mr. Washington, allow me to present Mrs.
Rust," (or Miss or Mr. Rust). If Mrs. Washington
extends her hand, Mrs. Rust takes it, but the latter
cannot make any advances to the distinguished or
elderly stranger.

If it is a formal reception, for those who are presented—and all guests are—only a greeting, and per-
haps the interchange of a sentence or two is possible.
If the introduction to a Mrs. Washington takes place
at an unceremonious party, her distinguished social
position or personal attainments give her the right to

open the conversation, but not the person presented. She has also the privilege of terminating an interview when she chooses to talk with another, or be silent. If she is accustomed to the graceful ways that prevail in good society, she does this in so gracious a manner that it is a captious person who is offended. No one is capable of being interested in all the world, much less of liking each person he or she meets. It is not a fault, although it may sometimes be a misfortune, that certain persons whom we would like to know feel little or no interest in us. Life would be an intolerable burden if we really made the acquaintance of every one whose manners or personality attracted us. A liberty to retain, as friends, such as are wholly sympathetic to us, according to our individual standards and tastes, is the charm of social liberty.

FORMAL AND INFORMAL ATTIRE.

A WOMAN who is acquainted with the requirements of good society in matters pertaining to the toilet, respects its canons. To be eccentric in dress, or even to be unusual, is impossible to her, as it would be, of course painful, if she has delicate sensibilities. The usual is the appropriate, also the most attractive at the time of its popularity. Properly clothed men and women are at their ease in any society. If a well-bred woman finds herself overdressed she is more uncomfortable than if too simply attired.

If the fact that she is overdressed is because she failed to recognize the informality of a social event, she is much more miserable than if her toilet had been less stately than the dignity of the occasion suggested. By her blunder, she has announced her unfamiliarity with prevailing usages.

By the well-bred woman is not meant the excessively vain one who never suspects herself of being too fine for any occasion. A man, unless he is a dandy or fop, never exceeds propriety in his attire or attempts very much ornamentation at any time unless

52

he is a foreign diplomat, or belongs to the army or navy.

Gentlemen and gentlewomen do not array themselves in garments that are not appropriate to the occasion. Thus much respect all guests at entertainments ought to pay their hostesses when an invitation is accepted. If appropriate toilets are beyond reach, a hospitality must be declined. This arbitrary law does not decide the quality of a fabric to be worn so much as its general effect, nor limit its age, so much as it requires it should be a formal dress. For example; a man must wear a dress suit at an evening party, or when calling and never by day, even at his own wedding. A frock coat, or cutaway, the former preferred, with light or dark trousers, is the visiting and afternoon or morning reception dress in good society. Gloves are always worn with the day costume, but in the evening, it is a matter of personal taste whether or not gloves in light colors shall be used. In case a guest is to dance, however, the wearing of gloves is *de rigueur*. Neckties are matters of fashion rather than of etiquette, although a little white cambric, silk, or satin tie is never out of style and never of questionable taste at a party or reception, day or night. For daylight any tie of prevailing mode is appropriate, a cheerful becoming color always preferred.

A tall silk hat is usual, though if it is to be left in the hall or dressing-room, its style is of small conse-

quence. Few men would carry a felt hat into a drawing-room, and the crush or opera hat appears to have
had its day in good society.   It was convenient in an
orchestra stall, at an opera or theatre, but as an orna-
ment for the hand of a man at an evening party, its
appropriateness, and especially its beauty, has always
been doubted, except by those who doted upon it.
Happily such have been few.   The approval of
society is never very far away from " sweet seasona-
bleness " and good taste, although obedience to its
requirements is seldom absolute and is not at all
regarded by certain rebels whom less amiable pens
mention as " costume cranks."

People who are always properly and tastefully
attired, win for themselves an especial admiration that
is not wholly unlike that which appreciators of perfec-
tion involuntarily give to a fine musician, or to one
who writes graceful verse.   It is the harmony of
external expression that obtains admiration.

Evening attire for women has its full and its demi-
toilet, the formality or informality of an invitation
deciding, or it should decide which raiment is appropriate.   If there is any doubt it is because the hostess
either desired to offer guests the liberty of choice in
dress, or she overlooked the fact that those whom she
addressed must necessarily judge of the dignity of the
event by the length of time intervening between the
issue of her cards and the evening of the party, quite
as much as from the style of the invitation.   If she did

not consider this fact, she can blame only herself if her entertainment is less brilliant and beautiful in costumes than she hoped and expected.

When there is a doubt regarding the ceremoniousness of an entertainment, it is more prudent to select a pretty demi-toilet than to appear in grand attire and with elaborate jewels.

Fresh flowers in discreet quantities and appropriate colors are always charming. With these tastefully disposed, according to prevailing modes, a gown that is less ceremonious and sumptuous in its texture or color than seems proper, is not in bad form at a party which was not announced by card as unmistakably formal or informal. [See "Good Form in Cards."]

Elderly men and women are allowed informalities that would be unpardonable in younger persons. Not that their attire in society is permitted to be less than dignified in style, but a high, closely buttoned coat or waistcoat and a gown closed at the throat with fully protecting sleeves are permissible, for health's sake, and because the dignity of age adds beauty and elegance to appropriateness.

Individuality in dress is not in bad form, provided it is individually suitable. Artistic effects are essentially in good form at a party, provided good taste is never violated.

Gowns that are superbly beautiful and pleasure-giving, when worn by those who are known to be rich, are wholly appropriate on grand occasions. The same toilet upon one, the weight of whose purse is an unsettled matter in the minds of fellow guests, produces a vague pain, or pity.

A woman who overweights herself with ornamentations, that is, one whose personality is lost beneath the sumptuousness of her raiment, so that only the impressiveness of her dress is recalled, might as well go into society by delegate or deputy, for all the admiration or appreciation she herself receives.

Gloves are worn by women through all entertainments except at dinners, where they are taken off when seated, and drawn on again at the end of the dessert, or as soon as the drawing-room is reached. At what Theodore Hook styled "perpendicular refreshments," one glove may be removed, should there be foods requiring use of the fingers. This, however, is a matter of personal preference and not of etiquette. One woman prefers risking a spot on the fingers of a glove to the unpleasantness of removing and putting it on again. It is not yet a custom, but in good society women with gloves reaching above their elbows have been seen unclosing a few glove buttons, and drawing out a thumb and finger, for use at a stand-up supper, and thereby saving their gloves without wholly uncovering their arms.

It is bad form to emphasize one's advancing age by an attire that is excessively or in the least needlessly grave, either in its form or color. Cheerfulness is due the young, and the absence of it in dress, simply because the afternoon of life is reached, is either an affectation or it is an evidence of morbid self-consciousness.

Rich jewels are never worn by gentlewomen in the street or indeed by daylight anywhere except at weddings or formal presentations. When diamonds glitter in a street car, the beholder involuntarily wonders if their wearers do not belong to families in which there are pawnbrokers.

It is indelicate and therefore bad form to dress with far greater elegance than a guest who has been invited to visit in the family, or to display personal belongings that compel unhappy comparisons of fortune between social equals. Exhibitions of costly adornments are only permissible between persons of known wealth, and even then some other amusement is preferable.

The truly courteous host does not forget that it is more gracious to accept hospitality than to bestow it, and that they who have the least abundance take it with the least pleasure, and often with the greatest reluctance. The recipient says in effect:

"I love you well enough to be indebted to you. This is the highest proof at my command."

Conventionality makes the host a servant to the guest, but the guest whose circumstances permit him no hope of returning courtesies in kind is most sensitive, a condition of mind which the finely bred host or hostess is not likely to overlook either at an evening entertainment, or during a visit of days. Especially is a well bred woman careful to wear simple gowns, that the guest staying in her house may not be made too painfully aware of the inattractiveness of her own raiment.

It is equally bad manners for guests to fail to make themselves as elegant as their resources permit, neither explaining nor apologizing for an unavoidable lack of prevailing mode in their wardrobe. To admit in words that one is restricted by poverty is to utter a complaint. A pleasant spirit adorns misfortune and compels admiration of a character and courage that bravely smiles in the face of want. The dignity of quiet endurance throws a glamour of beauty over threadbare garments and conceals their ugliness. Poverty is a crime only when it willingly offends good fortune.

SOCIAL AMBITIONS.

A DESIRE for position is almost universal among civilized people, and it need not be an unworthy ambition. Usually it is not, but the modes by which it is sought are too often ignoble.

One ambition is a craving to become fit companions of those who have honorably distinguished themselves. Both men and women eagerly desire to enter this charmed circle without considering whether or not their attainments, mental, material and personal, adapt them to its fastidious exactions of thought, habit and manner.

This class is catalogued among the "pushing." They usually rouse a fine scorn of their pretentious efforts; also a resolute determination to bar them out of the best society, which sentiment is certainly not the noblest. Considering the universal insistance of nature's first law—self-preservation—it is to be hoped that such as fail of maintaining their own ideas of generosity to all the world will be able to pardon themselves, if they keep the pushing man and woman down below, at the same time that they are intriguing to obtain higher positions, without properly cultivating themselves and making fitting adjustments of their habits to a higher social rank.

The question that most concerns the ambitious, who are usually also the earnest, the sincere and the educated, is, " Which is the highest social grade of which I, according to my own ideals of nobility of place and of refinement, am able to fill with honor and usefulness ? "

Having made a choice of purposes according to one's tastes, talents and circumstances, it is not good form to parade as one of another condition. Genuineness, representing the highest of its kind, can never be unrefined or ostentatious and vulgar.

A really intellectual public and an ultra fashionable one are too far apart in their aims and their pleasures for much satisfactory interchange of sociability. Of course they do touch each other in a common humanity, and here and there a person belongs to both classes. Sometimes there is a general commingling of courtesies, the fashionable individual feeling, though not mentioning the fact, his enjoyment of an implied compliment which he construes so that it means for himself, " I am also intellectual and accomplished, and consequently good company for the scholar."

Sometimes he is !

The scholar is not displeased now and then at being invited to be giddy and to meet society, these infrequent interchanges maintaining a mutual kindli-

ness, but establishing no real enlargement of hospitality in either sphere. This separation is well for both.
One keeps the world of industry astir, ministering to
its wants. The other learns the secrets of the uni-
verse and informs the fashionable world of as much of
its mysteries as amuse him, but keeps the best for his
own circle.

The two circles are too far apart in the qualities of
their social pleasures and each is too well adapted to its
own sphere to reasonably desire to intermingle inti-
mately. One is not above the other, unless intellectual
gifts or attainments that are consecrated to great
purposes, lift an individual or a set of individuals
higher than all their kind.

A thoughtful woman who has set a beautiful and
influencing mark upon the century said of another
woman who is a star in the fashionable firmament :

" She is too far above me in fashionable matters
and too far below me in intellectual ambitions and
interests, humane and practical. Why should we
waste our time, energies and sympathies upon each
other's purposes or tastes? We meet incidentally and
enjoy tidings from each other's realms, during which
times we are wholly unobservant of the fact that there
are antagonisms in our aims."

Life is made up of interdependencies that are most
useful, satisfying and harmonious, when there is no
attempt to make them " occupy the same place at the
same time."

This axiom is equally applicable to humanity in its social relations and positions. The robin might as well try to be a lark, and the goose a peacock as the man and woman who were born for practicalities to be miserably ambitious to become social butterflies. Charming as the latter are the former leave marks behind them that are not written in sand, a privilege denied to the butterflies.